Radiology of Haemophilic Arthropathies

Radiology of Haemophilic Arthropathies

Jenő Forrai, M.D.

Professor and Head, Department of Radiology
National Institute of Haematology and Blood Transfusion, Budapest

Technical assistance:

Éva Sümeghy

Radiology assistant

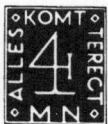

Springer-Science+Business Media, B.V.
1979

Referees:

F. Horváth, M. D.
Department of Radiology
National Institute of Occupational Health

Susan Csató, M. D.
Senior Lecturer
Department of Orthopaedics
Semmelweis University Medical School

Translated by

Anna Jánossy, M. D.

English translation edited by

E. Farkas, M. D.

The distribution of this book is handled by the following team of publishers:

for the United States and Canada

Kluwer Boston, Inc.
160 Old Derby Street
Hingham, MA 02043
USA

for all other countries

Kluwer Academic Publishers Group
Distribution Center
P.O. Box 322
3300 AH Dordrecht
The Netherlands

for Hungary, Albania, Bulgaria, China, Cuba, Czechoslovakia, German Democratic Republic, Democratic People's Republic of Korea, Mongolia, Poland, Roumania, Soviet Union, Democratic Republic of Vietnam, and Yugoslavia

Akadémiai Kiadó
1054 Alkotmány u. 21.
Budapest
Hungary

1st edition 1976
2nd revised, enlarged edition 1979

© Springer Science+Business Media Dordrecht 1979
Originally published by Akadémiai Kiadó, Budapest in 1979
Softcover reprint of the hardcover 2nd edition 1979

Joint edition published by
MARTINUS NIJHOFF PUBLISHERS
P.O.B. 566, 2501 CN The Hague, The Netherlands
and
AKADÉMIAI KIADÓ
1054 Alkotmány u. 21, Budapest, Hungary

ISBN 978-94-017-6461-2   ISBN 978-94-017-6600-5 (eBook)
DOI 10.1007/978-94-017-6600-5

Contents

Foreword

The use of potent coagulation factor concentrates has dramatically changed the clinical picture and the life expectancy of haemophiliacs. The aim of well-organized care of haemophiliacs is to prevent not only life-threatening bleeding episodes, but also the development of disabling arthropathies. In spite of numerous effective drugs and the beneficial effect of early synovectomy, haemophilic arthropathy will long remain a crux of everyday practice.

Based on 10 years' experience at the National Institute of Haematology and Blood Transfusion, this volume presents a detailed description of the X-ray morphology of haemophilic arthropathy. The rich series of illustrations should serve for guidance in diagnostics and differential diagnostics, and will provide help in establishing the stage and in estimating the prognosis. It will be of interest to all physicians engaged in the care of haemophiliacs.

Susan R. Hollán, M. D.

Corresponding Member of the Hungarian Academy of Sciences,
Professor of Haematology,
Director of the National Institute of Haematology and Blood Transfusion

Acknowledgements

I gratefully acknowledge the help of all those who have contributed to this monograph. First I wish to acknowledge the help of Professor Susan Hollán, Corresponding Member of the Hungarian Academy of Sciences, Director of the National Institute of Haematology and Blood Transfusion, Professor of Haematology at the Postgraduate Medical School, Editor-in-chief of *Haematologia*, an international quarterly, who provided us with the most modern equipment and has been interested in, and encouraged, our work throughout.

I wish to thank Professor I. Simonovits, Director General of the National Blood Transfusion Service, Director of the Department of Social Medicine, Semmelweis University Medical School, President of the National Committee of Haemophilia, for his continuous interest and help.

I am deeply indebted Ms. Éva Sümeghy for technical assistance, for preparing the radiographs, and for her help in getting this volume ready for the press.

I am indebted to Dr. Gy. Feszler, Head of the Surgical Department of the National Institute of Haematology and Blood Transfusion, Dr. G. Králl, Head of the Haemophiliac Care Centre and Dr. Susan Elődi, Head of the Laboratory of Blood Coagulation, for their friendly cooperation.

I wish to thank Mr. F. Ruzsmolnár for his excellent photographic assistance. A note of thanks is due to Dr. Anna Jánossy, the translator.

The Author

Introduction

In the last ten years many new and effective antihaemophilic therapeutics have been discovered and introduced. The therapeutical achievements have raised an active interest in the therapy of haemophilia [1–6]. Naitonal societies of haemophilia have been organized, which have launched programmes to rehabilitate haemophiliacs and promote their adaptation to social life [7–23].

In August 1975 a Symposium of the European Section of the International Society of Haematology discussed in detail the treatment and care of haemophiliacs in various countries. In Sweden [24] the ratio of haemophiliacs to the male population was 1 : 15,000. Between 1931 and 1975 the incidence of haemophilia — calculated for 5-year periods — remained practically unchanged. In the 284 registered families haemophilia A occurred in 77% and B in 23%. The number of haemophilia patients was 557/436 haemophilia A and 121 B. Of the haemophilia A cases 40% were severe, 18% moderate and 41% mild. The distribution was similar for haemophilia B. Eight and 10% of the severe haemophilia A and B patients, respectively, had factor VIII inhibitor. Prophylactic treatment of 4–18-year-old boys abated severe haemophilia to the moderate degree. In the past few years, owing to the use of antihaemophilic concentrates, factor VIII inhibitor has raised a problem ever increasing in importance, and immunological investigations have been initiated on a wide scale to tackle this problem [25].

At the time of the Symposium 429 haemophiliacs were registered in Greece [26]. In Italy [27] the incidence of haemophilia was 835 among 53 million inhabitants. In Spain [28] the number of recognized cases was 1172. In the FRG [29], among the 65 million inhabitants, 3000 cases were registered, and the number of haemophiliacs unregistered was estimated to be another 3000. In France [30] 2800 cases of haemophilia, including 2000 severe cases, were registered; of these 80% had haemophilia A and 20% had haemophilia B. In England [31] 1625 patients were registered, indicating that together with the unregistered cases the incidence of haemophilia was 3–6 per 100,000 population. In Spain 2–3, while in the U.S.A. 9 haemophiliacs were registered per 100,000 population. In England, the ratio of haemophiliacs was much lower over the age of 20 than under this age, indicating that before antihaemophilic theraphy was introduced the life-span of haemophiliacs had been much shorter than that of the general population.

In Hungary, the care of haemophiliacs is the responsibility of the National Institute of Haemotology and Blood Transfusion. As the head of the X-ray Department of this Institute I have had the opportunity of observing all cases of haemophilia treated at the Institute during a period of ten years (about 200 haemophiliacs). In 97 cases a detailed X-ray analysis was made. Most patients were regularly checked, hence we were able to follow the course of their illness from the radiological aspect.

This large patient population was studied in detail from the point of view of haemophilic arthropathies. Our motive for choosing this subject had been the increasing significance of haemophilia, since, due to the use of effective antihaemophilic concentrates, the average life-span of the patients increases [32–39], and the intracerebral [40] and other fatal haemorrhages can be favourably influenced. Thus, more and more patients grow up and reach a stage of the illness when the number and intensity of bleeding episodes decrease. By this age, however, most patients are severely handicapped by progressive arthropathy [41, 42]. This is the reason why recently surgeons have also become interested in this problem [43–53]. Since 1968 Italian surgeons have attempted to correct the arthropathies by synovectomy. Good results as regards reduction of bleedings and relief of pain have been reported [54–58].

In Hungary the organized care of haemophiliacs started in 1950. A National Committee of Haemophilia was established in our Institute in 1972, with Professor I. Simonovits as Chairman. The programme launched by the Committee included the drafting of the basic principles of haemophiliac care and the ways of organizing this work [59–67]. The Committee coordinates the research and organizational activities of the subunits. The number of haemophiliacs in Hungary is estimated at as high as 1000; of these about 400 are registered.

The history of medicine is rich in descriptions of haemophilia [68–69]. The disease had been recognized in ancient times already [70–73].

In 1803 Otto [74] and in 1872 Legg [75] reported that haemophilia was frequently associated with arthropathies. König's publication in 1892 [76] was the first to show that these arthropathies were due to intraarticular bleedings. This author distinguished three stages in the course of the disease. He gave a detailed description of haemophilic arthropathies, and his statements are still valid. Although many workers have tried to modify König's classification, the three stages he established have remained a firm basis for further studies.

The first stage, haemarthrosis, is an acute haemorrhage with swollen joints, pain, and limitation of function as characteristic features. No bony alterations are demonstrable radiographically. The second stage, panarthritis, is characterized by lesions of the synovial membrane, articular capsule, cartilage and the juxtaarticular area of the bone. The third stage, regression, is characterized by progressive deformities, ankylosis and contracture.

From the radiological aspect, König's first stage is characterized by the symptoms of acute haemarthrosis. These are easily recognizable and do not differ from those of haemarthrosis or hydrops of other origin.

As to the incorrect concept of the "specific intensity increase" of periarticular soft tissues occurring in stages 1 and 2 that has been widely accepted, a detailed discussion will follow below.

14

The symptomatology of stage 3 is likewise poor. Subsequent to panarthritis, the bone structure shows the picture of chronic atrophy, and fibrotic or, exceptionally, osseous ankylosis is found.

The actual osteoarticular process, panarthritis, is characterized by a wide variety of pathological, radiological and morphological features. It starts with the appearance of a fine marginal erosion subsequent to a few episodes of bleeding and comes to an end when the joint has been totally destroyed. In principle, we agree with König in that, though very long and variable, panarthritis is a single continuous pathological process. Nevertheless, for pratical reasons it is necessary to subdivide it into shorter periods, i.e. stages which are more uniform from the morphological aspect [77, 78].

Our knowledge of the histological features of the disease is poor. This is partly because it occurs rarely, and partly because it is hazardous to perform biopsy in haemophiliacs. The few available postmortem data mostly describe the late stage of regression, in which the less characteristic degenerative alterations are predominant [79–81]. Even today, the most valuable data are obtained from synovectomies, performed with protective AHG substitution, and not from postmortem findings.

The role of coagulation factors and the genetic aspects of the disease are not treated in the present monograph, and the reader is referred to the rich literature of these subjects [82–90].

The basic radiological findings in haemophilic arthropathies are well known [91–110]. However, the large number of cases in our material has provided an exceptionally good opportunity for making fresh observations and drawing additional conclusions [111].

In our opinion, a new survey on the radiomorphology of haemophilic arthropathies, published at a time when physicians are making ever growing efforts to combat this disease, will attract interest.

Statistical Data
and Basic Considerations

In the following, representative statistical data from our Haemophiliac Care Centre are presented.

The data of 77 consecutive cases have been processed from six aspects:

1. Age distribution
2. Type of haemophilia
3. Age at the first bleeding episode
4. Site of the first haemorrhage
5. Affected joints
6. Bleedings in other organs

Age distribution

It should be noted that our Institute has no paediatric department. Haemophiliacs under the age of 10 years are generally treated in children's hospitals. Most of our patients were between 20 and 40 years of age. These decades are critical from the

Age (yr)	No. of cases
0–10	3
11–20	18
21–30	24
31–40	18
41–50	9
51–	5
Total	77

point of view of the individual's whole life; this is the time when most people embark upon a career and start a family. Increased responsibility may be associated with emotional strain and a risk of bleeding episodes. Later on the frequency of bleedings is lower, and up to the present the average life-span of haemophiliacs used to be shorter, which also explains the low number of cases.

Type of haemophilia

The ratio of haemophilia A to B (5 : 1) is in agreement with the internationa average.

	No. of cases	Per cent
Haemophilia A	64	83
Haemophilia B	13	17
Total	77	100

Age at the first bleeding episode

In 2 of the 77 cases the age at which the first bleeding was observed was unknown. In 36 cases, i.e. in about half of the patients, the first haemorrhage occurred in the first two years of life and in 61 of the 75 cases it occurred below seven years of

Age (yr)	0	1	2	3	4	5	6	7	8	9	10–14	15–19	>20
No. of cases	16	20	9	2	5	9	—	1	1	—	7	3	2

age. Although in the early school-years bleedings occur frequently, the stress of schoolwork itself does not increase the frequency of the first symptoms.

In cases when the first haemorrhage occurs at a later age the symptoms are in general mild, and usually the further episodes are moderate in both frequency and severity.

Site of the first haemorrhage

Injury or haemarthrosis occurred in half of our cases (each in 18 cases). The type of injury and the site of the first episode of bleeding are more or less characteristic of the age of the patient at the time of the first bleeding. Under the age of 2 years, in 8 cases bleeding of the gingiva called attention to haemophilia, while in one case paracentesis performed at 3 months of age. In infants starting to walk, injury of the head, face and nose is rather frequent. The first manifestation often follows tonsillectomy or tooth extraction from the age of 5 to 6 years on. However, in extremely mild cases the disease may remain undiscovered until a tooth extraction over 20 years.

Affected joints

The following distribution was found in the 77 cases analysed:

Knee	Ankle	Hip	Elbow	Shoulder
82	41	22	54	12

The side of the affected joint was not registered. The order of frequency is in agreement with other published statistics: knee, elbow, ankle.

Bleedings in other organs

Naturally, in our patients bleedings also occurred in other organs, not just in joints. These included subcutaneous haematomas, fractures of extremities, gastrorrhagia, haemorrhage following gastric resection, epistaxis, gingival haemorrhage, intra-abdominal bleeding, etc. Nephrorrhagia occurred in 28 of the 77 cases. Although it is generally known that haematuria is common in haemophiliacs, this surprisingly high incidence suggests that renal manifestation of haemophilia deserves special attention.

Intracerebral haemorrhage occurred in 3 cases. In 2 of these no sequelae were observed, in one case repeated bleeding episodes led to the manifestation of epilepsy. Four of our patients had epilepsy without any previous history of intracerebral bleeding. In these cases the epilepsy may be attributed to previous micro-haemorrhagic processes without any clinical symptoms.

Stages of Haemophilic Arthropathy

As stated above, haemophilic arthropathy is a single, long process which starts as an acute intraarticular haemarthrosis and eventually leads to disabling regression through several episodes of bleedings, destruction of cartilage and degenerative changes of the subchondral bony tissue [112–122]. Its course is slow and progressive, although not without episodes of relative comfort, and there are no specific clinical, pathomorphological or radiological signs that would allow the distinction of characteristic stages of the disease. Nevertheless, for practical reasons, some sort of staging becomes necessary to characterize the patient's condition. In the present work we do not wish to critically analyse the various attempts at staging that have been undertaken, and adapt König's classical stages [76] which, despite their obvious shortcomings, still appear to be superior to subsequent classifications.

A dividing line cannot be drawn between acute haemarthrosis (stage 1) and panarthritis (stage 2), since the two conditions are frequently present concurrently and also because there is no specific radiological sign which would allow such a distinction. In principle, the first radiomorphological signs of panarthritis are changes in the epiphyseal contours. However, it is a long process from the first signs to the manifestation of unambiguous marginal erosions and subchondral lesions.

It would be an even more difficult task to delimit panarthritis from regression. Although these stages differ remarkably in their classical traits, the transition from one to the other lasts several years, and sometimes staging is only possible by determining the predominance of the radiological signs of one or the other condition. Although the entire process will in the following be discussed divided into stages, their frequent overlapping is not left out of consideration.

The general features described in the different stages of haemophilic arthropathy naturally vary in the individual joints. This is due to the anatomical and statical characteristics of the different joints. Therefore the special symptomatology of the individual regions will be discussed separately.

Acute Haemarthrosis

General clinical, pathological and radiomorphological aspects

Intraarticular haemorrhage occurs in all severe cases of haemophilia when the serum level of factor VIII is below 1%. Ali et al. [35], in a study of 210 haemophiliacs, found intraarticular haemorrhages in 196 cases (93%). Favre-Gilly [123] found haemarthrosis in 94% of 130 cases. Haemarthrosis generally appears in the early years of life [124]. Thomas [125] reported ankle haemarthrosis in a 3-month-old infant. In 89% of our own patients the first haemarthroses occurred under the age of 10 years. Lyon-Smith [126] reported a 70% manifestation below 2 years.

The first episode of haemarthrosis occurs very rarely over the age of 20 years. Any joint may be affected, the most frequent being those of the knee, elbow and ankle. Our own experience [111] is consistent with the data published by the Nuffield Orthopaedic Centre (Oxford) [127]. In 113 haemophiliacs treated between 1966 and 1969, haemarthrosis was found in 151 knees, 109 elbows, and 75 ankles. In other joints bleeding was less frequent. Nine wrists, 8 shoulders, 5 feet and 5 hips were affected. Jordan [46] recorded haemarthrosis in 56 cases. The order of the sites of the first manifestations was as follows: knee (97), elbow (72), ankle (52), shoulder (16), hip (16) and wrist (15).

It is generally accepted that articular haemorrhage is initiated by microtraumas which would be of no consequence in subjects with normal blood coagulation. This view is supported by the fact that the knee, elbow and ankle joints are injured the most frequently. However, some other joints, e.g. the temporomandibular articulation and the interphalangeal joints of hands and feet, are also frequently injured owing to their special functions and superficial topographies. Nevertheless, haemorrhages occur much less frequently in these joints. Thus, the possible role of some specific morphological or functional features of these joints must be postulated, which have so far been overlooked.

The clinical picture of acute haemarthrosis is characterized by pain and swollen joints. The intensity of the symptoms depends on the degree and rate of bleeding. Bleeding is generally assumed to be arterial. The articular capsule, being tense, causes pain which does not cease even during rest. Relief from pain indicates that bleeding has stopped.

De Andrade et al. [128] have demonstrated that filling of the knee joint with saline causes acute pain and limitation in function.

Distension of the capsule depends, beside the extent of haemarthrosis, on the degree of arthropathy. Recurrent haemarthroses result in a fibrous thickening of the capsule; hence, the capacity of the joint will be reduced.

Haemarthrosis may last for hours or for days. It is more likely to recur in affected joints than in intact ones.

Though the disease had been recognized thousands of years ago, our knowledge of its pathology is still limited. Surgical intervention in the affected joints had been avoided until recent years, and postmortem observations were also scarce because, the cause of death being usually not in direct connection with arthropathy, the joints were not examined in detail. Only few data have been obtained from animal experiments.

Basic information may be obtained from the works of Freund [129] and Key [130]. Freund made postmortem studies [129, 131], while Key [130] published the histological findings he obtained in a patient. Their observations and conclusions were practically identical.

The earliest sign of haemorrhage is microbleeding in the synovum mainly from the synovial villi. Blood then penetrates the articular cavity, and, in addition, an exudate rich in leukocytes, and later containing also macrophages, appears. The synovial villi show hypertrophy owing to epithelial proliferation, an overgrowth of fibrotic tissues and lymphocytic plasma cell infiltration. The fibrotic adhesion of the synovial villi is a significant feature of the process resulting in a narrowing of the joint cavity. After repeated bleeding episodes the adhesions inhibit articular function. It has been suggested that the traumatic detachment of these adhesive synovial villi may play a role in the recurrence of bleedings. In case of untreated haemophilic arthropathies blood clots loosely adherent to the synovial membrane and the neighbouring articular cartilage can be observed. Cicatrization, newly formed connective tissue, haemosiderin apposition in macrophages, and fresh small haemorrhagic foci are frequent and characteristic features of recurrent bleeding episodes.

Besides the adhesion of synovial villi, the thickening and progressive rigidity of the subsynovial tissue and articular capsule (particularly subsequent to repeated bleedings) play a role in the limitation of articular function. Synovial contracture often causes irreversible deformity.

In the early stage of haemophilic arthropathy, when the X-ray features are not pathognostic, clinical diagnosis is based on a triad, viz. coagulopathy manifested in boys; characteristic inheritance pattern; and deficiency of the relevant coagulation factor. At a more progressed stage many X-ray signs can be detected, none of which is pathognostic alone but the symptom complex is very characteristic and highly valuable in the rare cases when differential diagnostic problems occur. The X-ray signs have been reviewed recently by Middlemiss [132], Moseley [95], Boldero and Kemp [133], etc.

Haemophilia is a rare disease. According to Biggs [134], among 100,000 subjects 2 to 4 are affected. In Sweden (Ramgren [135]) and in Denmark (Sjolin [136]) 1 newborn male of 7000 newborns was found to be affected by haemophilia. In spite of its rareness, haemophilia is of great medical, social and economic [137] importance, as the treatment of haemophiliacs is a complex task for hospitals. Team work is necessary for comprehensive therapy, which is only possible in regional centres. Ali et al. [35] have recently discussed the importance of organizing regional centres.

Recently a follow-up of patients treated in regional centres has been performed with the aim of clarifying whether there is any significant difference in the X-ray course between cases of haemophilic arthropathy treated in regional centres on the one hand, and untreated cases, on the other. The data which have emerged are not suitable for drawing final conclusions.

Acute haemarthrosis causes distension of the capsule and oedema of periarticular tissues. Initially no bone lesions are present. The blood is totally absorbed and the joint recovers wholly within a few weeks. After recurrent bleedings, however, a chronic inflammation of the synovial membrane develops, revealed on the X-ray as the thickening of the capsule and synovium. This sign is made even more conspicuous by an unusually strong atrophy of the periarticular tissues. This condition cannot be distinguished radiologically from chronic synovitis of other origin (tuberculosis, rheumatoid arthritis).

Many communications have reported on the increased radiodensity of the periarticular soft tissues, presumably due to the large amount of haemosiderin impregnating them. The case of Freund [129, 131] in which he performed parallel radiographic and histological investigations is often quoted. He clearly demonstrated a decreased radiotransparency of the thickened tissues. Freund attributed this phenomenon to an increased iron content. He reported a 75% iron content in the ash of the thickened tissue. However, this latter statement has been questioned by others [138]. Freund's concept will be discussed in the chapter on panarthritis.

The radiological picture of acute haemarthrosis is dominated by the increased articular volume, which is especially conspicuous on comparative films. A widened soft tissue shadow is visible; consequently, the affected joint appears to be underexposed in comparison with the contralateral joint. (If the layer thickness of the swollen joint is taken into account before exposure, the normal joint will appear overexposed on the comparative film.) When X-ray pictures of cases of contracture either due to acute pain or occurring as a late manifestation are analysed similar technical problems will arise.

Another radiological sign indicating acute haemarthrosis is the widening of the joint space. Articular cartilages are forced apart by blood penetrating the joint space. The mode of dislocation is characteristic of the affected joint. The most striking and characteristic changes can be seen in the knee and shoulder joints.

An increased growth rate of the affected epiphyses in children with haemophilic arthropathy is a further sign that has repeatedly been dercribed. In spite of this, its possible pathognostic use has not been mentioned in the literature. This disorder is easily recognizable in the stage of panarthritis in children, sometimes soon after the first few haemarthroses which have not caused any visible destruction. It is worth mentioning that even atrophy may occur in children simultaneously with accelerated growth. This disproportionate epiphyseal growth can only be evaluated in comparative pictures. For this purpose the joints should be positioned symmetrically with great care before exposure. This is not an easy task when an arthropathic joint is to be compared with an intact one; an asymmetric posture due to contracture may mislead the observer. Sometimes ossification centres appear earlier in the affected joint than on the intact side. Later, the epiphyses of the affected joint are larger and develop faster than those on the opposite side. However, eventually, the affected joint does not overgrow the normal size. In fact, some authors have observed a premature termination of longitudinal growth and a premature osseous fusion of the epiphyses. The direct cause of the increased growth rate is, supposedly, the continuous hyperaemia accompanying chronic inflammation [139]. This suggestion is supported by the occurrence of an increased rate of epiphyseal growth in other chronic inflammatory processes [140].

Characteristic features of individual joints

Lower extremities

Arthropathic processes in the lower extremities are the basic cause of long-term crippling in haemophiliacs. The most severe lesions occur in the lower extremities, mainly in the knees and also frequently in the ankle joints. The hips are affected less frequently and less severely.

Knee

Acute haemorrhage results in swelling of the knee and an increase in its circumference. Accordingly, a widened soft tissue shadow is visible in the radiographs. The affected joint appears to be underexposed on comparative films which also differ in the quality of contrasts. The articular space is filled with fluid more or less evenly, forming a ball-like intumescence. In some cases an unusually large amount of blood is accumulated in the suprapatellar bursa, hence, the picture is dominated by the widening of the soft tissue shadow on the anterior surface of the distal third of the femur. The joint surfaces are forced apart by the haemorrhage producing an increased distance between the femoral and tibial articular surfaces. In younger patients this process is more intensive, in older patients it is limited by the rigidity of the tissues. Detachment also depends on the intensity of previous episodes: recurrent bleedings result in a fibrotic, inflexible, less distensible articular capsule, holding the joint surfaces rigidly.

The patella is more likely to get dislocated. Its anterior dislocation is due to the fluid accumulated between the patella and the femur. Sometimes an extreme dislocation occurs, accompanied by a lateral subluxation of 2 to 3 cm. This picture is highly characteristic of excessive haemarthrosis.

Ankle

The ankle joints are the third in the order of frequency among the sites of haemophilic arthropathy. However, the alterations are usually not as severe as in the knees. The reason for this seems to be the more restricted functional mechanism of this joint and the protective role of the ankle bones.

The first episode of bleeding often occurs in early childhood. The soft tissue changes characteristic of haemarthrosis are associated with a widening of the talotibial space. The talocalcaneal space may also be widened.

We have often observed a developmental anomaly of the ankle joint, which, to our best knowledge, has not yet been reported by others. The distal epiphysis of the tibia is abnormally shaped: it is gradually, but markedly, tapering in a mediolateral direction, sometimes to such an extent that it appears triangular because the articular surface meets the ossification line at an acute angle. In the frontal view the joint space is oblique in a lateral-proximal to medial-distal direction instead of being horizontal. The anomaly is compensated by a characteristic feature of the trochlea tali: its lateral half is larger, and also higher, than its medial half. In spite of this, the anomaly appears to play a role in the marked pes valgus, very common in haemophilia. In some cases it is accompanied by hypoplasia of the medial malleolus.

The primary cause of this complex anomaly is, in our opinion, an early atrophy of the distal epiphysis of the tibia which carries the weight of the whole body and is thus compressed.

Hip

The hips of haemophiliacs are affected less frequently. The onset of the procees is difficult to determine as the hip is deeply embedded in soft tissues, thus, its characteristic swelling may escape attention. To our best knowledge, no X-ray pictures have been published demonstrating the characteristic widening of the joint space. The slight early atrophy is hardly demonstrable because of the intensive scattered radiation. Hence, the diagnosis of haemarthrosis needs a thorough physical examination even if the basic illness and the complaints are known.

There are two further disorders worth mentioning in haemophilic arthropathy of the hip.

First, coxa valga occurs more frequently in haemophiliacs than in normal subjects; sometimes it is associated with hypoplasia of the acetabulum and femoral head. This characteristic feature which sometimes cannot be distinguished from congentital dislocation of the hip is well known in the literature and has been explained in many different ways. The data available at present fail to provide a solution of its aetiology. We support the suggestion that dysplasia of the hip joint and consequent coxa valga are due to subnormal functional load on the affected extremity due to the severe arthropathy of the knee and ankle joints. Similar deformities may develop after poliomyelitis and cerebral palsy. At the same time, some of our patients with serious knee deformities had no similar alterations in their hips.

Secondly, the sterile osteonecrosis of the femoral head, the so-called Perthes–Legg–Calvé–Waldenström disease, is worth special mention. The basic process is identical with the course in patients without coagulopathy (manifestation at the same age, i.e. 4 to 8 years, the same course and the same final outcome). The eventual deformity is a mushroom-like flattening of the head of the femur associated with coxa vara or coxa plana. This phenomenon seems to be explainable by the specific topography of the joint. Until the appearance of the ossification centre the femoral head consists of a cartilaginous substance with bradytrophic metabolism. Simultaneously with the appearance of the ossification centre, blood vessels penetrate the substance, ensuring a direct blood supply of the osseous tissue. Before the growth of the bones has come to an end, the growing substance of the epiphysis is exclusively supplied by the blood vessels coming directly from the joint cavity, as there is no blood supply either from the diaphysis or from the metaphysis at that time. The ramus acetabuli, a branch of the obturator artery (from the internal iliac artery) enters the hip joint through the acetabular notch and reaches the head of the femur through the ligament of the latter. The intraarticular section of these blood vessels is compressed by the haemarthrosis and the compression may severely disturb the blood circulation leading to necrosis of the ossification centre in the head of the femur. It may seem controversial that despite the coarse sclerotic fragmentation and shrinkage of the ossification centre, the joint surface is intact and smooth. The explanation is that the cartilaginous cover is not affected by the pathological process: the subchondral bony substance necrotizes, while the cartilaginous substance shows no trophic disorder, and after the regeneration of the bone adapts to the new formation. The size of the radiological joint space is normal, indicating that the chondral substance is intact. It is worth special attention that in haemophiliacs the regeneration of the osseous substance after Perthes' disease is identical with the regeneration in patients without coagulopathy; during recovery one would expect the regeneration of blood vessels to lead to intraosseous bleedings and to formation of cysts in the severely damaged tissue structures. However, no primary intraosseous haemorrhage occurs in these cases and even after Perthes' disease, alterations characteristic of the stage of panarthritis occur only if the cartilaginous cover has been damaged by repeated episodes of bleeding or by synovitis.

The course of haemophilic arthropathy in hips affected by Perthes' disease clearly indicates that the typical epiphyseal changes do not in general result from primary intraosseous haemorrhage, but from a degenerative process accompanying the destruction of the chondral substance.

Absence of the lateral part of the femoral head is a characteristic alteration we have frequently observed. A part of the head of the femur appears to be cut off flush with the cranial lateral ridge of the acetabulum. The radiographic contour is generally intact, distinct, only the adjacent bone is slightly rarified. This disorder is usually associated with dysplasia of varying degree. Besides the theoretical possibility of dysostosis as a pathogenetic factor, the lack of weight bearing and thus absorption due to inactivity may be considered.

The above-described changes might suggest an association of other inherited anomalies with the genetic deficiency of coagulation factors. This concept, however, still remains to be supported. A report of Putman et al. [141] has raised the possible existence of an inherited lung anomaly: of the 33 haemophiliacs examined by them radiologically 14 showed anomalies of lung blood vessels.

Upper extremities

In contrast to the statical function of the lower extremities, the function of the upper extremities is dynamic. In spite of the difference in function, haemophilic arthropathy is in many respects similar in the upper and lower extremities. This supports the concept that statical and dynamic microtraumas play an identical role in the manifestation of haemophilic arthropathies.

In the upper extremity, too, the three chief joints play a dominant role, whereas the smaller joints are much less frequently affected.

Elbow

The most significant alterations are found in the middle joint of the upper extremities, i.e. in the elbows. Obviously the dynamic strain is the most intensive in this joint.

The pathology of the haemophilic elbow is extremely varied, complex, and polymorphous, particularly in the stage of panarthritis. This is due to the complexity of the normal anatomy of this joint. It, in fact, consists of three differently functioning joints. The most important of these is the humeroulnar articulation between the trochlea humeri and the incisura trochlearis ulnae. The humeroradial articulation is formed between the capitulum humeri and the head of the radius. The proximal radioulnar articulation is formed between the circumference of the head of the radius and the incisura radialis ulnae. The humeroulnar articulation is a cylindrical joint, the humeroradial articulation is a spheroid one, whereas the proximal radioulnar articulation is a rotary one. The main function of the joint is the movement in the humeroulnar articulation: the main ridge of the incisura semilunaris ulnae moves in the groove of the trochlea humeri permitting of extension and flexion.

The patient with haemarthrotic elbow is forced to hold his arm at an angle of 120° because the distribution of the articular fluid and capsular tension determined by the balanced state of the muscles are optimal in this position, which means that pain is also the most tolerable. Fusiform swelling of the periarticular soft tissues is well visible. The X-ray picture shows, besides the forced position of the joints, an increased distance between the osseous articular surfaces in the humeroradial and humeroulnar joints. Distension of the radioulnar joint does not occur because of the tight intraosseous syndesmosis (membrana interossea antebrachii).

Shoulder

The haemarthrosis of the shoulder joint is poor in clinical symptoms and physical signs. The joint is deeply embedded in the shoulder muscles, hence, the degree of swelling is sometimes difficult to estimate. The subjective symptoms are naturally similar to those experienced in other joints.

In some cases the X-ray picture shows a widened joint space due to the increased intraarticular pressure. This distension is, however, uneven: the head of the humerus is situated somewhat more distally, and the articular space is wider cranially. These are important characteristics to be kept in mind because the condition might easily be mistaken for subluxation.

The epiphysis of the head of the humerus is characteristically deformed. Its proximal segment remains intact while it is narrowed distally, assuming the shape of a parrot's beak. After ossification has been completed, the head of the humerus is deformed, the epiphysis appears to be dislocated distally and the condition of humerus varus develops. This anomaly seems to be basically similar to the deformity of the distal tibial epiphysis described above.

Panarthritis

General aspects

According to König's classification the second stage of haemophilic arthropathy is panarthritis. The picture is characterized by changes in the synovial membrane, articular capsule, articular cartilage and in the juxtaarticular areas of the bone. The disease affects the tissues of the joints in various sites and by various mechanisms. This explains the extraordinary richness, complexity, and often individual divergence of the radiomorphology of this condition.

The blood vessels supplying the articular tissues are compressed by the increased intraarticular pressure, a consequence of haemorrhages [142, 143]. This plays a role in the manifestation of the first symptom, a slight diffuse osteoporosis. Loss of calcium is particularly striking in epiphyses of the long tubular bones which have not yet fused. Naturally, inactivity also plays a substantial role in the development of atrophy [144].

Increased pressure also results in erosion and resorption of the subchondral osseous tissue. Thus, the bone at the joint margins may extend by as much as 1 cm, mimicking the osteophytes occurring in common arthroses. However, pathologically just the reverse happens: osteophytes are due to apposition, whereas pseudo-osteophytes are due to resorption. Erosion is mainly detectable in the proximal tibial and distal humeral epiphyses. In cases when the contours are indistinct, suspicion of caries sicca may arise. With progression of the process the hyperplastic synovial layer of the joint capsule plays the key-role in chondral and bone destruction.

An increased radiodensity of the synovial tissues [129, 131] was also often seen by us. However, we agree with Boldero [133] and Pohlenz [138] that this increase is only apparent. Similar periarticular density increase can be observed in other serious processes where no absorption of blood occurs and no iron is present (e.g. tuberculosis, rheumatoid arthritis). In our opinion, the relative increase in the density of the periarticular tissues is due to marked osteoporosis and muscular atrophy, besides the hypertrophy of the synovial layer.

As a result of repeated bleeding episodes and the progression of haemophilic arthropathy, the initially fine lesions become more and more striking.

Owing to the destruction of chondral tissue, the chondral space becomes narrow. On the subchondral bony surface fine unevenness is visible and its contour becomes irregular, wavy, and fragmented. Fine stair-step formations and fissures are seen. Later, cysts develop in the cancellous subchondral layer of the epiphysis. These cysts are initially few in number and have the size of a pin-head, but later they increase in number and appear like a string along the contour of the joint surface. Most of these formations are hazelnut-sized, but plum- or nut-sized cysts may also occur.

The origin of these cysts is a matter of dispute. Until recently is was generally assumed that they are due to primary intraosseous haemorrhage [145, 148]. Some authors attributed the cysts to subchondral bleedings [49]. In our opinion they are the result of a degenerative process. We base our opinion on the radiographic similarity of these cysts to the degenerative cysts found in common arthrosis. Furthermore, in most of our cases tomography revealed a communication between the cysts and joint cavity, analogous to the picture of degenerative cysts. Recent histological data also support their degenerative origin [150].

Schwägerl et al. [151, 152] reported interesing observations made while performing synovectomies. The chondral surfaces were damaged by repeated bleeding episodes, crater-formed defects reaching into the subchondral region were observed especially in the weight-bearing areas. The remaining cartilage was loosened, in some parts elevated and detached, due to the haematoma localized underneath.

Experimental evidence is also available as regards the pathomechanism of this process. Swanton [153] observed haemophilic dogs for eleven years. Besides the above-mentioned synovial and capsular alterations, he studied subchondral cysts, drawing attention to the fact that no sign of bleeding appeared in them. He concluded that subchondrial haemorrhages play no substantial role in the formation of these cysts. The articular cartilage showed hardly any alteration: its surface was dull, finely granulated and slightly loosened. Key [154], Soeur [155] and Rigal [156] failed to reproduce the changes of haemophilic arthropathy by the injection of blood into joints of healthy animals. Young and Hudacek [157] repeatedly injected blood into the knee joints of dogs over a period of one year. Six months later there was a moderate villous hyperplasia and 8 to 12 months later marked fibrosis of the capsule. No notable lesion was found in the articular cartilage. Wolf and Mankin [158] found that earlier authors could induce experimental lesions only in the synovial membrane and articular capsule without the other alterations characteristic of haemophilic arthropathy. Therefore, they injected blood into the knee joints of rabbits twice a day and the joints were studied for up to the eighth week after the start of injections. No change was detected in the microscopic appearance or in the metabolic activity of the articular cartilage. Finally, Hoaglund [159] succeeded in reproducing synovial and cartilaginous changes characteristic of haemophilic arthropathy. He injected the knees of puppies with 1 to 4 ml blood six times a week. Among his observations a yellow pigmentation of, and fibrillar changes in, the cartilage deserve mention. His findings are inconsistent with Lack's view [160], who suggested that the cartilage is damaged by plasminogen activated by a cytokinase of leukocyte origin. In Hoaglund's experiments r-aminocaproic acid, a potent inhibitor of plasminogen activation, did not prevent the cartilage from being destroyed. Other proteolytic enzymes, however, might be present in the hypertrophied synovium which could cause degeneration of chondromucoprotein. Luscombe [161] has described such enzymes in the synovial membrane in rheumatoid arthritis. Fibrinolytic inhibition might even promote cartilage destruction via the mechanism fibrin → granulation tissue → arthropathy.

As regards the relationship between cartilage destruction and cyst formation, it seems to be of interest that in our large patient population no cysts were ever seen in cases with intact articular surfaces. They were, without exception, associated with other morphological alterations. However, the other lesions described above often occurred without cysts. This characteristic pattern of the symptoms and the dynamics of X-ray morphology may enable us to draw conclusions on the patho-mechanism.

The increased intraarticular pressure compressing the subchondral layer and the cysts produce marked reactive, mainly subchondral, sclerosis in the epiphysis.

This phase of panarthritis is highly variable. The growth of the epiphyses is rapid due to the synovial hypervascularization and the hyperaemia accompanying chronic inflammation. Consequently, the affected epiphyses are enlarged and their structure is loose. In the subchondral area and around the cysts, on the other hand, marked sclerosis dominates the picture. The articular space is narrowed, the joint surfaces are fragmented with pseudoosteophytes on their edges.

Wood et al. [77] evolved a very detailed score system for characterizing the progress of haemophilic arthropathy: thickening or calcification of the periarticular soft tissues, 1 point each; narrowing or widening of joint space due to haemorrhage, 1 point; enlargement of epiphysis, 1 point; osteoporosis: mild, 1 point; severe, 2 points; few (1 to 4) erosions, 1 point; >4 erosions, 2 points; few (1 to 4) cysts, 1 point; >4 cysts, 2 points; osteoarthritis: mild, 1 point; severe, 2 points; thickening of synovium, 1 point (this is not directly observable on the X-ray, only its consequences); finally Harris' line, 1 point. In our patients this latter occurred rarely, probably due to climatic differences. A point of dispute in this system is the separate listing of osteoarthritis, as most of the listed symptoms are parts of the osteoarthritis syndrome. Possibly, the authors thought, first of all, of pseudo-osteophytes when writing osteoarthritis. In this case it would be advantageous to substitute pseudoosteophytes for osteoarthritis in the scoring system. Wood et al. themselves admit it as a deficiency of their system that acute and chronic symptoms have not been separated. However, they claim that acute and chronic symptoms are often observed together. Most acute haemarthroses occur in joints with radiologically demonstrable chronic lesions.

This very careful attempt to classify cases has shown that even such a detailed scoring system meets serious difficulties. To mention but some of these: (a) evaluation of cysts is performed without accounting for their size; (b) the limit of 4 is arbitrary – why do 5 small cysts represent a more serious condition than 3 or 4 large ones, particularly if the cysts may range from pin-head to plum in size; (c) another source of error is the subjectiveness of differentiating between slight and severe cases of osteoporosis or osteoarthritis; (d) epiphyseal enlargement is variable, the terms "enlarged" or "not enlarged" are not sufficient for determining the condition.

It is worth drawing attention to the difficulties inherent in analysing the case history and clinical picture. Most haemarthroses occur at such an early age that the patient has no memories of them. Furthermore, haemarthroses are also different in severity. Thus, it would be to the purpose to establish criteria for the degree of haemorrhage, which again would be a difficult task.

Characteristic features

Lower extremities

Knee

In the initial stage of panarthritis either atrophy or overgrowth of the epiphysis of variable degree may be observed. Later, chondral tissue is destroyed and a fine unevenness and fragmentation of the subchondral bone contour appear. Resorption all around the subchondral area of the tibia results in the characteristic picture of pseudoosteophytes. Bone resorption also occurs in the subchondral marginal area of the femur. However, here the topographical situation is somewhat different: the chondrous cover of the femur is curled slightly upwards in all directions, thus also laterally. Resorption takes place under this cover and, therefore, ram-horn-shaped pseudoosteophytes are formed.

Subsequently, subchondral cysts appear. Cyst formation seems to be the most marked in the proximal epiphysis of the tibia. Innumerable lens- or pea-sized cysts are visible, some may reach the size of a plum. Many of them communicate with the articular space, as shown radiologically. The articular surface is pitted above areas where a large cyst or many small cysts develop. We wish to emphasize repeatedly that subchondral cysts have never been seen is cases of radiologically intact subchondral bone contours. The single cysts are outlined by a thin sclerotic border, but in the tibia and in parts of the femur, where mechanical stress is maximal, coarse diffuse eburnation occurs subchondrally.

The widening of the intercondylar notch was considered pathognostic for a long time. Jupe [162] attributed this lesion to haemorrhage at the site of attachment of the cruciate ligament. Also Johnson et al. [163] and Moseley [95] consider the deepening and widening of the intercondylar notch characteristic and suitable for the differentiation of haemophilic arthropathy from rheumatoid arthritis. Boldero and Kemp [133], on the other hand, did observe this symptom in rheumatoid arthritis. Then, in 1969, Bohrer [164] reported on a case of tuberculous synovitis with a pronounced widening of the intercondylar notch. In this case, that of a 12-year-old Negro girl who had suffered from intermittent pain in her right knee for three years, also marginal erosions were detected in the distal part of the femur and in the proximal part of the tibia. Based on X-ray findings the author assumed a coagulopathic origin. However, biopsy showed synovial tuberculosis.

This was a case of basic importance. Tuberculosis of the knee may start as a primary bone process or may start in the synovium. Synovial tuberculosis may extend, but not inevitably, to the bone. If the process is confined to the synovium, X-ray findings will be characteristic of chronic synovitis, irrespective of its origin. If the synovial membrane penetrates the intercondylar notch under the patella, an erosion may develop either in the notch or marginally on the uncoated bone surface.

Discussing the differential diagnostics of haemophilic arthropathy tuberculosis is usually not mentioned in connection with the widening of the intercondylar notch. On the other hand, this alteration was mentioned by Pugh [165] and Ganguli [166] when discussing the tuberculous alterations of the knee.

Thus widening of the intercondylar notch may be the result of haemophilia, rheumatoid arthritis or tuberculosis if any of these diseases is accompanied by chronic synovitis.

A technical detail needs mentioning here. For projecting the intercondylar notch, the patient must lie prone, his knee flexed at an angle of 120°, while the central beam is perpendicular to the cassette. A similar position is required for the anterior–posterior projection if there is a slight contracture of the knee; in this case, too, the intercondylar notch is well visible. We wanted to clarify whether in haemophilic arthropathies this position might explain the widening of the intercondylar notch. However, the phenomenon was also visible when the limbs were fully extended during exposition.

The patellar lesions are principally the same as those seen in affected articular surfaces in general. The cartilage is worn away and the joint surface is fragmented and uneven; later small subchondral cysts appear in the slightly sclerotic area.

Besides the above changes, the so-called squared off patella is particularly characteristic. In advanced haemophilic arthropathies the distal apex is flattened. Initially, the patella participates in the accelerated growth, later, however, its distal apex is flattened and the characteristic squared off patella develops. According to Jordan [46] this is the consequence of premature cessation of growth, particularly in the lower segment of the patella. This view is not easy to prove, as in the distal part of the patella ossification centres occur but seldom. Caffey [167], reviewing the development of the patella, suggests the possible appearance of irregular ossification centres. He presents the X-ray picture of the patella of an 11-year-old boy showing a small ossification centre. Schinz [168] displays a drawing of a similar patella, the distal part of which is designated "lower paranucleus". Köhler and Zimmer analyse these variations in great detail in their handbook [169]. In the opinion of these authors a small isolated ossification centre at the lower apex of the patella is a regular feature, but it is visible for a very short time only. They demonstrate three such cases. In the atlas of Matzen and Fleissner [170] a persistent apophysis in the distal apex of the patella of a 20-year-old male is shown. Sinding-Larsen [171] and Johannsohn [172] also reported a transitory ossification disorder in the distal apex of the patella. In their case cortical erosion and a separate bone plate were visible on the distal apex. This disorder is only observable in young people, and is assumed to be the consequence of an overstrain in the patellar ligament due to excess in football or dancing. The condition is listed among sterile osteochondronecroses in text-books. Uniform interpretation of this morphological picture meets difficulties as it may occur with or without clinical symptoms. Our opinion may be summarized as follows. The ossification centre at the distal apex is a regular feature or at least a frequent phenomenon, however, due to its early fusion, it can be observed for a short time only. Its persistence is a rare phenomenon. Before fusion, sterile necrosis may occur, similarly to the process in Schlatter–Osgood's disease. An X-ray picture may in itself be insufficient for establishing whether in a given case this isolated ossification centre may cause complaints.

Accepting Köhler's [169] opinion offers a reasonable explanation of the squared off patella. Hyperaemia associated with chronic inflammation stimulates the fusion of the apophysis, thus growth of the bone is prematurely completed. This is a modern version of Jordan's earlier hypothesis, in the light of recent literature.

Whatever the pathomechanism of the phenomenon, it is obvious that such a well-defined form is extremely rare in other atropathies, thus it is more or less pathognostic for haemophilia. Grokoest et al. [173] and Chlosta et al. [174] encountered this disorder in a case of juvenile rheumatoid arthritis. This agrees with our observations. We have never seen this peculiar disorder in cases when haemarthroses appeared at a relatively advanced age, but it was common in cases in which the first episodes occurred in early childhood. Hence, continuous hyperaemia at an early stage of development seems to be a prerequisite of squared off patella.

Ankle

In the stage of panarthritis massive subchondral sclerosis of the ankle joint is seen with few but large cysts, in contrast, e.g. to the knees, where small cysts frequently occur. The cysts in the talus are generally large, and the trochlear articular surface above them is broken down.

Hip

The classical symptoms of panarthritis are less severe in the hip joints than in either the knees or ankles. Fragmentation and stair-step formation on, and a few small cysts beneath, the articular surface are well visible. Large cysts usually communicate widely with the articular space. Owing to the statical situation, frequently small isolated fragments appear on the proximal arch of the femoral head, i.e. osteochondritis dissecans indicating severe destruction also develops.

Upper extremities

Elbow

The elbow joint is highly suitable for following up the maturation of the bone system as its numerous ossification centres appear at different ages: that in the capitulum of the humerus at 2 years of age, while those in the head of the radius, in the medial epicondylus, and in the trochlea at 5 to 6, 6 to 9 and 8 to 10 years, respectively. Those in the lateral epicondylus and in the olecranon appear at 13 years and that in the apex of olecranon somewhat later. The fusion of the ossification centres takes place from the 14th year on.

The stimulating effect of inflammatory hyperaemia on growth and maturation is particularly striking in the elbows. The progression of the process can be measured on comparative X-ray pictures of children's elbows. On the affected side the ossification centres appear earlier, or are larger, than on the intact side.

The occurrence of a supratrochlear foramen, a characteristic regional anomaly, is particularly striking in the stage of panarthritis. In the literature this anomaly is considered a variation. It often shows familial clustering and is in general bilateral. In some mammalian species it is regularly present. Schinz [175, 176], who studied the anomaly in detail, believes that it is a phylogenetical remnant.

The anatomical explanation of the anomaly is as follows. Under physiological conditions the coronoid fossa and the olecranon fossa situated opposite each other are separated by a thin bone plate, which is missing in this variation. Hence, a foramen of lens- or nut-size is formed.

We have observed a strikingly high frequency of this anomaly in the arthropathic elbows of haemophiliacs. A hereditary origin connected with that of coagulopathy in these patients may arise. This presumption would be supported by the familial cumulation of the variation in non-haemophiliacs. However logical this assumption seems to be, we firmly deny it. According to our own experience, the anomaly may be unilateral, and it always occurs in the more severely affected joint. Therefore, the supratrochlear foramen in haemophiliacs is due to repeated intraarticular bleedings and the consequent increase in intraarticular pressure, resulting in the resorption of the membrane separating the two fossae. Sometimes a reactive marginal sclerosis develops on the ridge of the resorbed intraosseous membrane. The whole process is analogous to the widening of the intercondylar notch in knee.

The intraosseous membrane as a locus minoris resistentiae may cause further characteristic alterations, as we have seen in our studies. Normally, on the surface of the trochlear notch of the ulna three is a dorsovolar crest, which is functionally a conductor: fitting into the notch situated similarly in the middle of the humeral trochlea, it prevents lateral slipping of the two joint surfaces. Due to the destruction of the cartilaginous surface, the epiphyseal bony substance is denuded, hence, it is less resistant to microtraumas. In advanced haemophilic arthropathy the conductor ridge of the olecranal notch actually saws the trochlea in two and penetrates into the coronoid and olecranon fossae, or into the supratrochlear foramen. Hence, a pseudojoint develops between the trochlear notch and the conductor ridge, sometimes even sclerosis occurs. The changes in the humeroradial joint are also characteristic. As the longitudinal growth of the radius is hindered in the proximal direction by the humerus, the head of the radius is characteristically deformed: its disc flattens and bulges radially, sometimes overgrowing the opposite humeral joint surface by as much as 1 cm; the capitulum of the humerus is generally flattened.

The protuberance of the trochlea penetrates the ulnar part of the olecranal articular surface so deeply that a pseudoarticulation is formed between the distal contour of the ulnar epicondylus of the humerus and the ridge of the olecranal joint surface.

In one of our cases a striking evidence of constant axial compressure was observed, viz. a characteristic fatigue fracture was seen under the head of the radius at the level of the proximal tubercle of the radius.

Arthropathic lesions may also develop in the proximal radioulnar articulation. Osteophytes on the distal ridge of the ulnar articular surface of the radius are characteristic in such cases.

Pseudoosteophytes are frequently formed on the volar and dorsal ridges of the capitulum humeri. Sometimes the original joint surface is undermined to such an extent that only a peg-like formation is seen in the place of the capitulum.

Subchondral cysts occur in all parts of the elbow, whereas giant cysts are characteristic of the olecranon.

Shoulder

Alterations in the shoulder joint characteristic of panarthritis are generally moderate. Unevenness of the articular surface is initially manifested over the distal third of the articular surface of the head of the humerus, later it may extend to other parts. Sometimes coarse alterations are found in the glenoid fossa. Characteristically situated subchondral cysts are seen, larger cysts being mostly sited near the proximal edge of the anatomical neck. As a result of resorption, pseudoosteophyte is formed along the distal contour of the anatomical neck. Rarely humerus varus occurs.

Wrist

Manifestation in the wrist is common, however, the changes are generally not pronounced and, if so, not characteristic. The picture is strikingly similar to common arthrosis. In some cases the two conditions differ only in the multiple occurrence of small cysts in haemophilic arthropathy.

Inside the carpus lesions mainly occur on the radial side. In mild cases arthropathy can be detected in the articulations of the radius and navicular bone. Often the plain X-ray picture only displays a flattening of the radial contour of the navicular bone, while tomography may reveal the fine unevenness of the contour already at this stage. Later on, the radionavicular space becomes narrowed, the lunate bone is deformed and subchondral cysts appear. Characteristic, coarse arthropathy is frequent between the navicular bone and the greater and lesser multangular bones, but it may also occur in the articulation between the lesser multangular and the 2nd metacarpal bones. These alterations occur in the stage of panarthritis. The stage of haemarthrosis of the wrist has not been discussed in the present work separately as it has no typical radiological features and the clinical picture is identical with that of other haemarthroses. In the stage of regression, too, no specific signs can be distinguished apart from slight atrophy.

The carpometacarpal articulations are frequently, whereas the metacarpophalangeal and the interphalangeal articulations very rarely affected.

The regional anomaly of a pea-sized transparency occurs in the area between the navicular, capitate and lesser multangular bones. This is a rare condition and, according to some authors, it corresponds to the cartilage form of an accessory bone, the os centrale carpi.

Regression

General aspects

The basic radiological signs of König's phase of regression are as follows. The bones forming the joint are very porotic. The uniform porosis, which in stages 1 and 2 is manifested as acute atrophy and in which the epiphyseal structure almost disappears, progresses in stage 3 into a picture characteristic of chronic atrophy. The spongy bone structure can be identified, although the bone trabeculae are considerably rarified and thickened and are situated as required by functional adaptation. The compact substance is thinner and the tubular bones are narrowed and hypoplastic along their entire length. With the destruction of the cartilage, the chondral space is narrowed, sometimes it is only virtual, but osseous ankylosis is rare. The narrowing of the articular space is morphologically different from that seen in the stage of panarthritis. While in the latter stage it is uneven and variable, in regression it becomes more uniform, as a result of restorative processes, indicating that the previously severely eroded subchondral bone contours have more or less regenerated, and a smooth, continuous contour has newly formed. In our opinion, it is very important and characteristic of this stage that the numerous subchondral cysts formed in the 2nd stage slowly disappear, giving place to a chronic atrophic structure. The intensive subchondral sclerosis also disappears. Pseudoosteophytes are not so prominent now because the eroded areas have been partly filled up. However, the coarse bone destruction cannot be entirely restored, thus, the epiphyses remain more or less deformed.

Characteristic features

Knee

The joint space is strongly narrowed and the bone structure displays chronic atrophy. The epiphyses are deformed due to a severe destructive process. The previously eroded contours become distinct again.

Hypoplasia of the fibula may be striking. Osseous ankylosis occurs but rarely. Tibiofemoral ankylosis is less frequent than patellofemoral ankylosis. Characterstic subluxation often develops, the tibia being subluxated dorsally to the femur.

Ankle

There are no specific characteristics of this joint in the stage of regression. It seems worth mentioning that, for statical reasons no doubt, the rarified bone trabeculae were strikingly thick here. In neglected cases pes equinus developed.

Hip

Since there is no severe destruction in the hip joint in the stage of panarthritis, the alterations in the 3rd stage are also moderate. Even fibrotic ankylosis is a rare phenomenon. Degenerative arthrotic lesions may appear at a relatively early age.

Elbow

The changes in the elbow joint agree with the general characteristics of the regression stage. Ankylosis does not develop, the affected epiphyses are deformed.

Shoulder

Haemophilic arthropathy usually manifests itself in this joint at a relatively late age. The whole course is slow and prolonged, and thus the stage of regression is rarely observed. Besides the general features, humerus varus is a common phenomenon.

Other Characteristic Conditions of Haemophiliacs

Pseudotumour

Bleeding episodes — independent of arthropathy — are frequent in the musculoskeletal system. In the majority of cases, haemorrhages occur intramuscularly, and their site, size and extension are sufficiently revealed by physical examination. However, the situation is entirely different when the bony substance is damaged by the haemorrhage. Bone destruction may be due to a primary intraosteal or subperiosteal haemorrhage, yet in most cases the pressure of intramuscular bleeding or haematoma accounts for bone usuration [180]. Since the first description of pseudotumour [181], 80 cases [182] have been reported. Pseudotumour may occur in the long tubular bones, first of all in the lower extremities. Over one third of the cases have been reported in the femur, somewhat less than one third in the pelvis. Generally, the lesion is related to trauma. The pseudotumour often appears as an irregular calcification or ossification in the soft tissue shadow, surrounded by bone erosion and bone regeneration. The radiological picture often indicates an extraosteal origin.

The small bones of the hand and foot, too, are often affected. These display an expansive cystic growth starting from the spongy substance, associated with secondary cortical destruction. Pseudotumour occurs relatively often in the calcaneum [183].

The differentiation of these bone changes may meet difficulties, even if the basic illness is known. Due to the similarity to osteosarcoma, pseudotumour is sometimes designated as haemophilic pseudosarcoma. A case was reported [184] of a haemophiliac with Ewing sarcoma, which was misdiagnosed as a haemophilic pseudotumour. Chondromas, cysts, fibromas, osteomyelitis, tumour metastases, aneurysmal cysts, giant cell tumours, plasmocytomas, echinococcosis, coccidioidomycosis and histiocytoma may also cause differential diagnostic problems.

Bone fractures

In haemophilia care centres it is well known that bone fractures occur much more often in haemophiliacs than in the normal population. This is due to several factors. The tubular bones forming arthropathic joints are poor in calcium, often hypoplastic and, due to the arthropathic process, they may show chronic atrophy. Thus, these bones are fragile. The movement of these joints is hampered, therefore, the patient when falling down is unable to protect himself. In addition, for psychological reasons, haemophiliacs often want to prove that they are as good, or even better, at games and sports as healthy children, therefore, they are heedless to danger. Roentgenograms of bone fractures of haemophiliacs are often suggestive of an insufficient treatment. Is the bone fracture treated at a department where specialized knowledge, practice and equipment are not at disposal, the patient may remain untreated as the medical staff knowing the basic disease will consider any surgical intervention too hazardous. The opposite, i.e. underestimation of the risk, may also happen, the patient is operated on without sufficient AHG protection. Both situations may result in unsatisfactory healing of the bone fracture, which occurs in nonhaemophiliacs extremely rarely. The duration of recovery, i.e. of callus formation, does not differ from the normal. Due to the lack of, or insufficient, reposition, enormous callus with extreme dislocation, shortening of the extremity and deviation of axis may occur. Supracondylar femur fractures are relatively frequent and characteristic in haemophiliacs. In the absence of dislocation and due to technical difficulties of X-ray caused by arthropathy this type of fracture may remain undetected in the slightly porotic bone.

Myositis ossificans

Calcification and ossification due to bleeding episodes are rare compared with the high incidence of intramuscular haemorrhages. Exceptionally bizarre heterotopic bone regeneration showing regular tubular bone structure may surround the hip joint [185]. In the literature 8 such cases have been reported; we found two among our patients. Figs 71b and c demonstrate the postmortem preparation of the hip joint of one of our patients.

Haematuria

Haematuria is a frequent, often recurring, symptom. Ramgren's [186] study of 176 Swedish haemophiliacs, and examinations performed in Oxford [187] indicate that this symptom follows haemarthrosis in the order of frequency. According to the statistics reported by the Hemophilia Society of the Netherlands [188], in 435 registered haemophiliacs followed up for 4 years, 3% of all the observed bleeding episodes were of urogenital origin. Radiological examination excluded any other origin of the bleeding (renal calculus, tumour, etc.) and coagulation tests confirmed haemophilia. The blood clot gives a negative shadow, and contrast urography may reveal moving pea- or bean-sized blood clots in the pyelon and calyceal trunks. X-ray examination reveals whether or not the blood clot has obstructed the kidney or whether the obstruction has ceased.

Gastrointestinal haemorrhages

Intramural bleeding is rare in the gastrointestinal tract; a few cases have been reported in the stomach, intestines and colon. Acute submucosal haemorrhage of the stomach appears clinically as an acute abdomen. X-ray reveals a large haematoma bulging into the gastric lumen [189]. Intestinal haematoma causes an irregular narrowing of the lumen, the haustration disappears, and the contours are indented, the haemorrhagic ileal loop is situated somewhat farther away because the thickened intestinal wall dislocates the narrowed lumen [190]. Larger haematomas produce a picture resembling a ladder due to plical swelling [191]. Melaena may be associated with this proces.. In extreme cases occlusive ileus may develop. As soon as the haematoma has been absorbed the symptoms gradually disappear.

Retroperitoneal bleedings

Retroperitoneal haematoma occurs rather frequently. If large enough, it appears as a soft tissue shadow with indistinct contour in the plain abdominal X-ray picture. Indistinct contour of the psoas muscle is a characteristic radiological sign. These haematomas may extend in various directions and may vary widely in size. A characteristic radiological sign of late complication is bone resorption in the area of the ilium, which, in fact, is a "bone cyst" or "pseudotumour". Sonography has been used in the past few years for accurate determination of the site and extension of such haematomas [192].

Intrapulmonary bleeding episodes and haemothorax

These are relatively rare complications. Intrapulmonary haemorrhages may occur in any part of the lung; these have no characteristic morphological features, although in some cases the intrapulmonary shadow is unusually intensive. Exceptionally, concurrent necrosis and cavitation may occur. The radiological picture of haemothorax does not differ from the generally known features of pleural exudations of other origin.

Neurological complications

Neurological complications may be due to intracranial haemorrhage, bleeding into the spinal canal or haemorrhage causing lesions of peripheral nerves. Naturally, invasive neuroradiological examinations can only be performed after sufficient preparation of the patient and if the factor level is ensured [193–195].

The Role of Radiology in Diagnostics and Care

Differential diagnosis of haemophilic arthropathy

The radiomorphological features described and analysed in the foregoing contribute to the differential diagnosis of haemophilic arthropathy. However, the general rule that all the X-ray signs may indicate several different pathological processes must be taken into account. Therefore, we stress that in spite of the detailed knowledge of X-ray morphology, X-ray pictures are always to be evaluated as part of the clinical picture and should be fitted into it, together with the physical and laboratory findings. Simultaneously, we wish to draw attention to some fundamental X-ray differential diagnostic problems, particularly as it may happen in spite of organizational efforts that it is the radiologist who first sees the patient, and he may have to decide on further examinations.

Let us take the commonly occurring case that a child falls down, hits his knee, which then becomes swollen. The practitioner sends the child to the X-ray department. Clinically the knee is swollen and is painful when moved, the X-ray displays an extended soft tissue shadow and a widened joint space.

Haemarthrosis cannot be differentiated from articular hydrops due to trauma or acute arthritis on the basis of radiological findings. The case history may reveal whether similar swelling has occurred in any of the child's joints. The first manifestation of haemophilia is rare over 20 years of age. If the history raises the slightest suspicion, coagulation must be examined.

In the stage of panarthritis the origin of the disease has generally been established due to the prolonged course of the process. Rarely, differentiation from tuberculous arthritis [164–166] and from progressive chronic polyarthritis [173, 177] may be necessary. Naturally, other chronic processes (diabetic or psoriatic arthropathy, ochronosis, etc.) may have similar features [178], moreover, at the peak of haemophilic panarthritis, when coarse reactive sclerosis, erosion of surfaces and marginal defects simultaneously occur, the bizarre picture is very similar to the polymorphism of tabetic and syringomyelic arthropathies [179].

Obviously, in most cases a correct diagnosis may be achieved by considering the changes described above. However, it cannot be verified without clinical and laboratory results.

The X-ray appearance of regression closely resembles the picture of healed tuberculous arthritis, but also that observed after all severe destructive processes of the joints. Furthermore, a similar picture may be seen in certain kinds of paralysis including poliomyelitis.

Radiology in haemophiliac care

Finally, the general principles of the radiological examination of heamophiliacs should be summarized.

Two basic types of X-ray examinations are performed: firstly, basic documentation, i.e. the total radiological status of the joints; secondly, occasionally performed examinations.

Under the age of 6, if there is an unambiguous family history and the typical clinical features are present, only the affected joint should be examined. In cases when the family history is unclear and clinical symptoms are obscure, all examinations usually performed in general osteoarticular diseases (rheumatic fever, acute leukaemia, etc.) should be carried out.

Over the age of 6, in cases of proved haemophilia a full X-ray examination is recommended as follows: anterior–posterior (A–P) view of both shoulders, hips, dorsovolar view of both wrists, A–P and lateral views of elbows, knees and ankles. Comparative examination is highly recommended.

In cases of recurrent haemarthroses when the basic documentation is available new pictures are unnecessary. Follow-up examination of joints frequently affected by haemarthroses should be made every 2 to 3 years. Naturally, when other alterations are suspected, such as fractures, X-ray examination is necessary.

Before surgical interventions – in the first place before synovectomy – a very careful X-ray exploration of the joint is to be carried out. Tomographic analysis revealing the exact state of the bone surfaces, further, the character and extent of the intraosseous processes are of great help to the surgeon.

Precise documentation of the X-ray condition of patients is an important part of haemophiliac care. However, considering the long duration of this disease, polypragmasy should be avoided.

Conclusions

Radiology plays an important role in confirming the diagnosis of haemophilia, in solving differential diagnostic problems, in the indication of surgical intervention and in the care of haemophiliacs. A detailed and accurate description of the X-ray symptomatology has been attempted in this monograph. We have also tried to fit the single radiomorphological signs into the entire, long pathological process.

We hope that this work will contribute to the endeavour of our Institute to participate effectively in the international efforts aimed at preventing haemophiliacs from being crippled.

References

1. Haemophilia prophylaxis. Editorial. *J. Amer. med. Ass. 212*, 2256 (1970).
2. Creveld, S.: Prophylaxis of joint hemorrhages in haemophilia. *Acta haemat. (Basel) 41*, 206 (1969).
3. Allain, J. P., Steinbach, M., Meunier, L., Muller, J. Y., Soulier, J. P.: Substitutive treatment of haemophilia "A" using a new factor VIII concentrate. *Nouv. Presses Méd. 5*, 1047 (1976).
4. Barthels, M., Gerstel, J.: Verlauf hämophiler Gelenkblutungen bei ambulanter Substitutionstherapie. *Dtsch. med. Wschr. 100*, 1523 (1975).
5. Schimpf, Kl., Fischer, B., Rothmann, P.: Die ambulante Dauerbehandlung der Hämophilie "A"; eine kontrollierte Studie. *Dtsch. med. Wschr. 101*, 141 (1976).
6. Aronstam, A., Arblaster, P. G., Rainsford, S. G., Turk, P., Slattery, M., Alderson, M. R., Hall, D. E., Kirk, P. J.: Prophylaxis in haemophilia: A double-blind controlled trial. *Brit. J. Haemat. 33*, 81 (1976).
7. Brinkhous, K. M.: *Hemophilia and New Hemorrhagic States*, University of North Carolina Press, Chapel Hill 1970.
8. Rizza, C. R., Biggs, R.: Haemophilia today. *Brit. J. Hosp. Med. 6*, 343 (1971).
9. Aszódi L., Szabó, Gy.: Haematológiai betegek gondozásának kérdései (Problems of care of haematological patients). *Haematologia Hungarica 3*, 153 (1963).
10. Brackmann, H., Egli, H.: Erste Erfahrungen in der Ausbildung Hämophiler in der Selbstbehandlung. *Hämophilie-Blätter 4*, 29 (1971).
11. Britten, A. F. H.: Haemophilic surgery. *Haemophilia research, clinical and psychosocial aspect. VIth Congress of the World Federation of Haemophilia.* Schattauer, Stuttgart–New York 1971.
12. Favre-Gilly, I.: Les hémophiles. *Réadaptation*. Numero spécial. *157*, 1969.
13. Franklin, F. J.: Trends in the treatment of haemophilia: patient–administered clotting factor program. *Haemophilia, reserach, clinical and psycho-social aspect. VIth Congress of the World Federation of Haemophilia.* Schattauer, Stuttgart–New York 1971.
14. Göbel, M., Schulz, R. D.: Möglichkeiten der Selbstbehandlung von Hämophilien. *Dtsch. med. Wschr. 15*, 37 (1972).
15. Green, D., Smith, N. J.: Haemophilia. Current concepts in management. *Med. Clin. N. Amer. 56*, 105 (1972).
16. Hirschmann, R., Itscoits, S., Shulman, N. R.: Prophylactic treatment of factor-VIII-concentrate. *Blood 35*, 189 (1970).
17. István, L.: Haemophiliás gyermekek gondozása (Care of haemophilic children.) *Orvosképzés 6*, 67 (1972).
18. István, L.: Haemophiliások sorsát befolyásoló medicinális és medico-szociális tényezőkről (On medical and medico-social factors concerning the fate of haemophiliacs). *Orv. Hetil. 113*, 3016 (1972).
19. István, L.: Adatok a haemophilia magyarországi gyakoriságához (Incidence of haemophilia in Hungary). *Dem. Sle. 1*, 1973.
20. Bidwelle, E., Dike, W. R.: *Treatment of Haemophilia and Other Coagulation Disorders.* Blackwell, Oxford 1966.

21. Landbeck, G., Kurme, A.: Aktuelle Probleme der ärztliche Versongung Hämophiler. *Fortschr. Med. 14*, 525 (1972).
22. Rák, K.: Haemophilia-syndroma. In: Braun, P. (ed.): *Ritka kórképek (Rare syndromes)*. Medicina, Budapest 1968.
23. Rosenthal, M. G.: *Management of Haemophilia*. The National Hemophilia Foundation, New York 1971.
24. Nilsson, I. M.: Management of haemophilia in Sweden. *Thromb. Haemostas. 35*, 510 (1976).
25. Ekert, H., Firkin, B. G.: Recent advances in haemophilia and Von Willebrand's disease (Editorial). *Vox Sang. 28*, 409 (1975).
26. Mandalaki, T.: Management of haemophilia in Greece. *Thromb. Haemostas. 35*, 522 (1976).
27. Mannucci, P. M., Ruggeri, Z. M.: Haemophilia care in Italy. *Thromb. Haemostas. 35*, 531 (1976).
28. Martin-Villar, J., Ortega, F., Magallon, M.: Management of haemophilia in Spain. *Thromb. Haemostas, 35*, 537 (1976).
29. Brackmann, H.-H., Hofmann, P., Etzel, F., Egli, H.: Home care of haemophilia in West Germany. *Thromb. Haemostas. 35*, 544 (1976).
30. Allain, J. P.: Management of haemophilia in France. *Thromb. Haemostas. 35*, 553 (1976).
31. Rizza, C. R.: The management of haemophilia in the United Kingdom. *Thromb. Haemostas. 35*, 559 (1976).
32. Editorial: Treatment of haemophilia. *Lancet II*, 648 (1973).
33. Landbeck, G., Kurme, A.: Die Hämophilie. Kniegelenk-Arthropathie. Ein Beitrag zur Behandlung von Kniegelenkblutungen und ihren Folgerständen. *Mschr. Kinderheilk. 118*, 29 (1970).
34. Ahlberg, A.: Treatment and prophylaxis of arthropathy in severe haemophilia. *Clin. Orthop. 53*, 135 (1967).
35. Ali, A. M., Gandy, R. H., Britten, M. I., Dormandy, K. M.: Joint haemorrhage in haemophilia: Is full advantage taken of plasma therapy? *Brit. med. J. 3*, 828 (1967).
36. Landbeck, G.: Therapie mit Faktor VIII und IX Präparaten. In: Pettenkofer, H. (ed.): *Gezielte Therapie mit Blutbestandteilen*. Lehmanns Verlag, München 1968.
37. Landbeck, G.: Häufigkeit und Schweregrade der Hämophilie. Entwicklung der Blutungs-symptomatik. In: Thies, H. A., Landbeck, G. (eds): *Hämophilie. XI. Hamburger Symposion über Blutgerinnung*, 1968. Schattauer, Stuttgart-New York 1969.
38. Deutsch, E.: Coagulopathien. In: Linneweh, F. (ed.): *Die Prognose chronischer Krankheiten*. Springer, Berlin-Göttingen-Heidelberg 1960.
39. Favre-Gilly, J., Hoen, J. P., Thouverez, J. P., Saint Paul, E.: Expérience de la chirurgie dans hémophilie. A propos de 220 interventions chez 136 hémophilies. *Anesth. Analg. Reanim., 32*, 591 (1975).
40. Friedman, H., Guerry, R., Wickins, R. H.: Intercerebral hematoma in a hemophiliac. *J. Amer. med. Ass. 215*, 791 (1971).
41. Abildgaard, Ch. F.: Current concepts in the management of hemophilia. *Semin. Hematol. 12*, 223 (1975).
42. Mackay, S. R.: Hemarthrosis (Discussion paper). *Ann. N. Y. Acad. Sci. 240*, 342 (1975).
43. Rothermel, J. E., Raney, Sr. R.: The change in prognosis in haemophilic arthropathy. *Sth. Med. J. (Bgham, Ala.) 62*, 1430 (1969).
44. Miller, E. H., Flessa, H. C., Glueck, H. J.: The management of deep soft tissue bleeding and hemarthrosis in hemophilia. *Clin. Orthop. 82*, 92 (1972).
45. France, W. G., Wolf, P.: Treatment and prevention of chronic haemorrhagic arthropathy and contractures in haemophilia. *J. Bone Jt Surg. 47B*, 247 (1965).
46. Jordan, H. H.: *Hemophilic Arthropathies*. Thomas, Springfield 1958.
47. Jordan, H. H.: Our present orthopedic management of haemophilia. In: Brinkhous, K. M. (ed.): *The Hemophilias*. University of North Carolina Press, Chapel Hill 1964.
48. Tarney, T. J.: *Surgery in the Haemophiliac*. Thomas, Springfield 1968.

49. Hubenstorf, H.: Die Gelenkskomplikationen der Hämophilie und ihre orthopädische Behandlung. *Wien. klin. Wschr. 80*, 139 (1968).
50. Buchner, H.: *Das Blutergelenk und siene Behandlung.* Enke Verlag, Stuttgart 1965.
51. Barta, O., István, L.: A haemophiliás haemarthros korszerű kezelésének 10 éves eredményei. Előadás a II. Magyar Haematológiai Napok ülésén (Ten years' results in modern therapy of haemophilic haemarthroses. Lecture presented at the IInd Hungarian Haemotological Congress), Pécs 1963.
52. Ahlberg, A.: Haemophilia in Sweden. VII. Incidence, treatment and prophylaxis of arthropathy and other musculo-skeletal manifestations of haemophilia A and B. *Acta orthop. scand., Suppl. 77* (1965).
53. Post, M., Telfer, M. C.: Surgery in hemophiliac patient. *J. Bone Jt Surg. (Boston) 57*, 1136 (1975).
54. Storti, E., Traldi, A., Tosatti, E., Davoli, P. G.: Synovectomy for hemophilic heamarthrosis. *Arthr. Found. Med. Bull. 11*, 21 (1970).
55. Storti, E., Traldi, A., Tosatti, E., Davoli, P. G.: Synovectomy in haemophilic arthropathy. A new approach to therapy and haemostasis. *Schweiz. med. Wschr. 100*, 2005 (1970).
56. Storti, E., Ascari, E., Magrini, U.: L'activité fibrinolytique dans la synoviale hémophilique. *Schweiz. med. Wschr. 102*, 1614 (1972).
57. Storti, E., Traldi, A., Tosatti, E., Davoli, P. G.: Synovectomy, a new approach to haemophilic arthropathy. *Acta haemat. (Basel) 41*, 193 (1969).
58. Storti, E., Traldi, A., Tosatti, E., Davoli, P. G.: Synovectomy for haemophilic haemar throsis. *Lancet II*, 572 (1968).
59. Simonovits, I., Králl, G.: A haemophilia gondozás helyzete Magyarországon (Haemophilic care in Hungary). *Transfusio 7*, 2 (1973).
60. Hollán, Zs., István, L., Feszler, Gy.: Medical organization of hemophiliacs in Hungary. *Bibl. haemat. (Basel) 26*, 153 (1966).
61. Simonovits, I., Hollán, Zs.: Praeventio a haematologiában (Prevention in haematology). *Orvosképzés 41*, 89 (1966).
62. István, L.: Adatok a haemophilia klinikumához, kezeléséhez és gondozásához (Data on the clinical manifestation of haemophilia, treatment and care of haemophiliacs). *Orv. Hetil. 112*, 3055, (1971).
63. Králl, G.: Haemophiliac care in Hungary. In: Deutsch, E., Pilgarstoofer, H. W. (eds): *Haemophilia.* Schattauer, Stuttgart 1971.
64. Simonovits, I.: Results in the care of haemophiliacs in Hungary. In: Mannucci, P. M., Randi, U., Di Giuliomaria, A. (eds): *Medical and Social Problems of Haemophilia in Europe and the Action of National Haemophilia Societies.* Fondazione Dell'Emofilia, Milano 1971.
65. István, L.: A haemophiliások rehabilitációja (Rehabilitation of haemophiliacs). *Transfusio 7*, 10 (1973).
66. Petrovan, O., István, L.: Adatok a haemophiliások személyiségképéhez (Data on the personality of haemophiliacs). *Transfusio 7*, 170 (1973).
67. Elődi, Zs.: Laboratóriumi módszerek vérzékeny betegek szűrővizsgálatára (Screening methods for the detection of haemorrhagic disorders). *Transfussio 7*, 210 (1973).
68. István, L.: A haemophiliával kapcsolatos kultúrtörténeti és történelmi adatok orvosi jelentősége (Medical importance of culture historical and historical data on haemophilia). *Transfusio 6*, 51 (1972).
69. Haefliger, H.: *Zur Geschichte der Hämophilie unter besonderer Berücksichtigung der Schweiz.* Baseler Beröffentlichungen zur Geschichte der Medizin und der Biologie, Vol. 28. Schwabe, Basel 1969.
70. Albukasin, K.: Liber theoreticae nec non practicae Alsaharavii 1519. Cit. by István [68].
71. Schloessmann, H.: *Die Hämophilie.* Enke, Stuttgart 1930.
72. Llopis, F.: *Hämophilie und ihre Behandlung (Wissenschaftliche Grundlagen).* Johann Ambrosius Barth, Leipzig 1929.

73. Rothschild, J.: Über das Alter der Hämophilie. Inaug. Diss. München 1882.
74. Otto, J. C.: An account of an haemorrhagic disposition existing in certain families. *Medical Repository 6*, I (1803).
75. Legg, J. W.: *A Treatise on Haemophilia.* H. K. Lewis, London 1872.
76. König, F.: Die Gelenkserkrankungen bei Blutern. *Volkmanns Sammlung Klinischer Vorträge 36* (1892).
77. Wood, K., Omer, A., Shaw, M. T.: Haemophilic arthropathy. A combined radiological and clinical study. *Brit. J. Radiol. 42*, 498 (1969).
78. István, L.: On the clinical manifestation of haemophilia, treatment and care of haemophiliacs. Thesis, Szombathely 1969.
79. De Palma, A. F., Cotler, J. M.: Hemophilic arthropathy. *Clin. Orthop. 8*, 163 (1956).
80. Rodman, G. P.: Some observation on experimental hemarthrosis and the pathogenesis of hemophilic arthritis. *Lab. Invest. 8*, 1278 (1959).
81. Brinkhous, K. M.: Hemophilia. *Clin. Pathol. 4*, 342 (1964).
82. Ala, F., Denson, K. W. E.: *Haemophilia.* Excerpta Medica, Amsterdam 1973.
83. Biggs, R.: *Human Blood Coagulation, Haemostasis and Thrombosis.* Blackwell, Oxford 1972.
84. Colman, R. W.: Immunologic heterogeneity of haemophilia. *New Engl. J. Med. 288*, 369 (1973).
85. Green, D.: Factor VIII (anti-hemophilic factor). *J. Chron. Dis. 23*, 213 (1970).
86. Ingram, G. I. C.: The genetics of clotting factor VIII. *Med. Lab. Techn. 28*, 76 (1971).
87. Mason, D. Y., Ingram, G. I. C.: Management of the hereditary coagulation disorders *Semin. Hematol. 8*, 158 (1971).
88. Ratnoff, O. D., Bennett, B.: The genetics of hereditary disorders of blood coagulation. *Science 179*, 1291 (1973).
89. Rizza, C. R.: The management of haemophilia. *Practitioner 204*, 763 (1970).
90. Stormorken, H., Owren, P. A.: Physiopathology of hemostasis. *Semin. Hematol. 8*, 3 (1971).
91. Stiris, G.: Bone and joint changes in haemophiliacs. *Acta radiol. 49*, 269 (1958).
92. Buus, C. E. P.: Articular changes in hemophilia. *Acta radiol. 16*, 503 (1936).
93. Steim, H., Doll, E.: Intraosseale Blutungen bei Haemophilie. *Fortschr. Röntgenstr. 91*, 746 (1959).
94. Fonio, A., Bühler, W.: Die röntgenologische Darstellung des Blutgelenks anhand von 136 Gelenksaufnahmen der Fonio'schen Sammlung. *Radiol. Clin. (Basel) 21*, 5 (1952).
95. Moseley, J. E.: *Bone Changes in Haematologic Disorders (Roentgen Aspects).* Grune and Stratton, New York–London 1963.
96. Favre-Gilly, J. E., Jouvet, M., Bétuel, H., Viret, J.: *Les données de la radiologie dans les séquelles des hémarthroses des genoux chez l'hémophile.* Masson et Cie, Paris 1961.
97. D'Alo, R., Pozzi, L.: Hemophilic arthropathy. *Minerva med. 52*, 1104 (1961).
98. Berg, C., Herzog, M.: Die verschiedenen Stadien des Blutergelenkes im Röntgenbild. *Fortschr. Röntgenstr. 65*, 126 (1942).
99. Canigiani, T.: Gelenkveränderungen bei Hämophilie. *Röntgenpraxis 2*, 511 (1930).
100. Cocchi, U.: Röntgendiagnosis der Knochenveränderungen bei Blutkrankheiten. *Fortschr. Röntgenstr. 77*, 276 (1952).
101. Davidson, C. K., Epstein, R. D., Miller, G. F., Taylor, F. H. L.: Hemophilia. *Blood 2*, 97 (1949).
102. Forfota, E.: Über die Gelenk- und Knochenveränderungen bei Blutern. *Röntgenpraxis 3*, 399 (1931).
103. Ghormley, R. K., Clegg, R. S.: Bone and joint changes in hemophilia. *J. Bone Jt Surg. 30/A*, 589 (1948).
104. Günsel, E.: Über krankhafte Veränderungen an Knochen und Gelenken bei Blutern. *Röntgenpraxis 14*, 81 (1942).
105. Holstein, J.: Die Gelenkveränderungen bei Hämophilie im Röntgenbild. Bericht über 30 Fälle. *Dtsch. Gesundh.-Wes. 15*, 2470 (1960).

106. Kuzmin, D. S., Tichomirova, T. I.: Voprosy rentgenodiagnostiki krovoizlijanij pri gemofilii. *Aktual. Vopr. Gematologii (Leningrad) 14*, 305 (1963).
107. Lampy, M.: L'aspect radiologique des ostéoarthropathies hémophiliques. *Bull. Soc. méd. Hop. Paris 58*, 45 (1942).
108. Newcomer, N. B.: The joint changes in hemophilia. *Radiology 32*, 573 (1939).
109. Reboul, J., Delorme, G.: Radio-diagnostic ostéoarticulaires dans l'hémophilie. *J. Méd. Bordeaux 132*, 293 (1955).
110. Webb, J., Dixon, A. S. J.: Haemophilic arthropathy. *Lancet II*, 1175 (1959).
111. Forrai, J., Feszler, Gy.: Az arthropathia haemophilica réteganalízise (Tomographic analysis of haemophilic arthropathy). Kongr. Suppl. 76. *Magy. Radiol.* (1968).
112. Ceaen, J.: Les hémarthroses hémophiliques. *L'hémophilie 29*, 5 (1963).
113. Chiari, H.: Die blutigen Gelenkserkrankungen. In: *Handbuch der spez. pathol. Anatomie und Histologie*. Springer, Berlin 1934.
114. Dubois, J. L.: L'ostéo-arthropathie hémophilique. *J. belge Méd. phys. rheum. 85*, 15 (1960).
115. Györgyi, G.: Haemophiliás csontelváltozások (Changes in the bones of haemophiliacs). *Magy. Radiol. 10*, 13 (1958).
116. Kuzmin, D. S., Klimenchenko, G. A.: X-ray diagnosis of hemophilic bleeding of various, localization. *XII. International Congress on Blood Transfusion*. Moscow, 17–23 August, 1969 Abstracts, p. 600.
117. Layani, F., May, V., Pelisson, J., Paquet, J.: Arthropathies hemophiliques. *Rev. Rheum. 26*, 463 (1959).
118. Novikova, E. Z.: Osteoarticular changes in hemophilia. *Vestn. Rentgenol. Radiol. 35*, 13 (1960).
119. Novikova, E. Z.: Changes in bones and joints in haemophiliacs. *XIIth International Congress on Blood Transfusion*. Moscow, 17–23 August, 1969. Abstracts, p. 599.
120. Reinecke-Wohlwill: Über hämophile Gelenkserkrankungen. *Langenbeck's Arch. klin. Chir. 154*, 425 (1929).
121. Tenberg, J. E., Ramgren, O., Plengiér, L.: Hemophilic arthropathy. *Acta rheum. scand. 6* 125 (1960).
122. Webb, J. D., Dixon, A. St. J.: Haemophilia and haemophilic arthropathy. An historical review and a clinical study of 42 cases. *Ann. rheum. Dis. 19*, 143 (1960).
123. Favre-Gilly, J.: Expérience de cinq ans du Centre Emile Remigy de Montain (Jura) pour Jeunes Garçons Hémophiles. *Hémostase 4*, 231 (1964).
124. Krause, W., Lasch, H. G.: Die Hämophilie. *Med. Klin. 64*, 367 (1969).
125. Thomas, H. B.: Some orthopedic findings in 98 cases of hemophilia. *J. Bone Jt Surg. 18*, 140 (1936).
126. Lyon-Smith, G. L.: Cit. by [133].
127. Duthie, R. B., Matthiews, J. M., Rizza, Ch. R., Steel, W. M.: *The Management of Musculo-skeletal Problems in the Haemophilias*. Blackwell, Oxford 1972.
128. De Andrade, J. R., Grant, C., Dixon, A. St. J.: Joint distension and reflex muscle inhibition in the knee. *J. Bone Jt Surg. 47-A*, 313 (1965).
129. Freund, E.: Die Gelenkserkrankungen der Bluter. *Virchow's Arch. path. Anat. 256*, 158 (1925).
130. Key, J. A.: Hemophilic arthritis (Bleeders' joints). *Ann. Surg. 95*, 198 (1932).
131. Freund, E.: *Gelenkserkrankungen*. Urban und Schwarzenberg, Berlin–Wien 1929.
132. Middlemiss, J. H.: Hemophilia and Christmas disease. *Clin. Radiol. 11*, 40 (1960).
133. Boldero, J. L,. Kemp, H. S.: The early bone and joint changes in hemophilia and similar blood dyscrasias. *Brit. J. Radiol. 39*, 172 (1966).
134. Biggs. R.: Thirty years of haemophilia treatment in Oxford. *Brit. J. Haemat. 13*, 452 (1967).
135. Ramgren, O.: A clinical and medico-social study of haemophilia in Sweden. *Acta med. scand.* Suppl. 379, III (1962).
136. Sjølin, K. E.: *Haemophilic Diseases in Denmark*. Blackwell, Oxford 1960.

137. Carter, F., Forbes, C. D., Macfarlane, J. D., Prentice, C. R. M.: Cost of management of patients with haemophilia. *Brit. med. J. 2*, 465 (1976).

138. Pohlenz, O.: Cit. by [133].

139. Cockin, J., Gilbert, M. (1972), cit. by [127].

140. Blount, W. P.: Unequal leg length. Instructional Course Lecture, American Academy of Orthopaedic Surgery, St. Louis *17*, 218 (1960).

141. Putman, Ch. E., Gamsu, G., Zinn, D., McLoud, Th.: Radiographic chest abnormalities in adult hemophilia. *Radiology 118*, 41 (1976).

142. Trueta, J.: The orthopaedic management of haemophilia. *Brit. J. Surg. 48*, 8 (1960).

143. Trueta, J.: The orthopaedic managemenet of haemophilia. *Proc. roy. Soc. Med. 55*, 1058 (1962).

144. Geiser, M., Trueta, J.: Muscle action, bone rarefaction and bone formation. An experimental study. *J. Bone Jt Surg. 40-B*, 282 (1948).

145. Steel, W. M., Duthie, R. B., O'Connor, B. T.: Haemophilic cysts. Report of five cases. *J. Bone Jt Surg. 51-B*, 614 (1969).

146. De Palma, A. F.: Hemophilic arthropathy. *Clin. Orthop. 52*, 145 (1967).

147. Jones, D. M.: Haemophilic blood cyst. *J. Bone Jt Surg. 47-B*, 266 (1965).

148. Bourdon, R., Bernard, J., Caen, J., Bard, M., Patrux, C.: Données évolutives des lésions ostéo-articulaires radiologiques de l'hémophile. *Sém. Hôp. Paris 58*, 2818 (1963).

149. Salerno, N. R., Menges, J. F., Borns, P. F.: Arthrograms in hemophilia. *Radiology 102*, 135 (1972).

150. Swanton, M. C.: *The Pathology of Hemarthroses in Hemophilia. Hemophilia and Hemophiloid Diseases. International Symposium*. Univ. of North Carolina Press, Chapel Hill 1957.

151. Schwägerl, W.: *Knochen-, Weichteil- und Gelenksveränderungen bei der Hämophilie A und B*. Facultas, Wien 1975.

152. Schwägerl, W., Niessner, H., Novotny, Ch., Thaler, E., Lechner, K.: Synovektomie zur Prophylaxe rezidivierender hämophiler Gelenkblutungen. *Dtsch. med. Wschr. 101*, 738 (1976).

153. Swanton, M. C.: Hemophilic arthropathy in dogs. *Lab. Invest. 8*, 1269 (1959).

154. Key, J. A.: Experimental arthritis. The reaction of joints to mild irritants. *J. Bone Jt Surg. 2*, 705 (1929).

155. Soeur, R.: The synovial membrane of the knee in pathological conditions. *J. Bone Jt Surg. 31-A*, 317 (1949).

156. Rigal, W. M. Cit. by Trueta J.: *Studies of the Development and Decay of the Human Frame*. Heinemann, London 1968.

157. Young, J. M., Hudacek, A. G.: Experimental production of pigment villo-nodular synovitis in dogs. *Amer. J. Pathol. 30*, 799 (1954).

158. Wolf, C. R., Mankin, H. J.: The effect of experimental hemarthrosis on articular cartilage. *J. Bone Jt Surg. 47-A*, 1203 (1965).

159. Hoaglund, F. T.: Experimental hemarthrosis. The response of canine knees to injections of autologous blood. *J. Bone Jt Surg. 49-A*, 285 (1967).

160. Lack, C. H.: Chondrolysis in arthritis. *J. Bone Jt Surg. 41-B*, 384 (1959).

161. Luscombe, M.: Acid phosphatase and catheptic activity in rheumatoid synovial tissue. *Nature (Lond.) 197*, 1010 (1963).

162. Jupe, M. H. In: Shanks, S. C., Kerley, P. (eds): *Text-Book of X-ray Diagnosis by British Authors*. Saunders, Philadelphia 1950.

163. Johnson, J. B., Davis, T. W., Bullock, W. H.: Bone and joint changes in hemophilia. *Radiology 63*, 64 (1954).

164. Bohrer, S. P.: Tuberculous synovitis with widening of the intercondylar notch of the distal femur. *Brit. J. Radiol. 42*, 703 (1969).

165. Pugh, D. G. Cit. by Bohrer [164].

166. Ganguli, P. K. Cit. by Bohrer [164].

167. Caffey, J., Schlesinger, E. R.: Certain effects of hemophilia on the growing skeleton. *J. Pediat. 16*, 549 (1940).
168. Schinz, H. R., Baensch, W. E., Friedl, E., Uehlinger, E.: *Lehrbuch der Röntgendiagnostik*. Thieme, Stuttgart 1952.
169. Köhler, A., Zimmer, E. A.,: *Grenzen des Normalen und Anfänge des Pathologischen im Röntgenbild des Skelets*. Thieme, Stuttgart 1967.
170. Matzen, P. F., Fleissner, H. K.: *Orthopaedic Roentgen Atlas*. Thieme, Stuttgart 1970.
171. Sinding-Larsen, M. F.: *Acta Radiol. 1*, 171 (1921/22). Cit. by [169].
172. Johannsohn, S.: *Z. orthop. Chir. 43*, 82 (1924). Cit. by [169].
173. Grokoest, A. W., Snyder, A. J., Schlaeger, R.: *Juvenile Rheumatoid Arthritis*. Little, Brown and Co., Boston 1962.
174. Chlosta, Eu. M., Kuhns, L. R., Holt, J. G.: The "patellar ratio" in juvenile rheumatoid arthritis. *Radiology 116*, 137 (1975).
175. Schinz, H.: *Fortschr. Röntgenstr. 29*, 193 (1922). Cit. by [169].
176. Schinz, H.: *Radiol. clin. (Basel) 14*, 19 (1945). Cit. by [169].
177. Martel, W., Holt, J. F., Cassidy, J. T.: Roentgenologic manifestation of juvenile rheumatoid arthritis. *Amer. J. Roentgenol. 88*, 400 (1962).
178. Teske, H. J., Siegenthaler, D.: Röntgendiagnose und Differentialdiagnose der alkaptonurischen Ochronose. *Fortschr. Röntgenstr. 102*, 689 (1965).
179. Porta, E., Sodano, A., Blasi, P., Fucci, G.: Semeiologia radiologica nella evoluzione clinica e nella terapia della osteoarthropathia emofilica. *G. ital. Chir. 26*, 3 (1970).
180. Ahlberg, A. K. M.: On the natural history of hemophilic pseudotumor. *J. Bone Jt Surg. 57*, 1133 (1975).
181. Starker, L.: Knochenusur durch ein hämophiles subperiostales Hämatom. *Mitt. Grenzgeb. Med. Chir. 31*, 381 (1918).
182. Hussey, H. H.: Hemophilic pseudotumor of bone. *J. Amer. med. Ass. 232*, 1040 (1975).
183. Hrodek, O., Tolarová Jaroslava, Snobl, O.: Hämophiler Pseudotumor im Calcaneus. *Folia heamat. (Lpz.) 101*, 654 (1974).
184. Gunning, A. J., Biggs, R., Macfarlane, R. G.: The surgery of haemophilic cysts. In: Biggs, R., Macfarlane, R. G. (eds): *Treatment of Haemophilia and other Coagulation Disorders*. F. A. Davis Company, Philadelphia 1966.
185. Hutcheson, J.: Peripelvic new bone formation in haemophilia. *Radiology 109*, 529 (1973).
186. Ramgren, O.: Haemophilia in Sweden. *Acta med. Scand. 171*, 237 (1962).
187. Rizza, C. R., Matthews, J. M.: Management of haemophilic child. *Arch. Dis. Childh. 47*, 451 (1972).
188. Veltkamp, J. J., Schrijver, G., Willeumier, W., van de Putte, B., van Dicjk, H.: Hemophilia in the Netherlands. *Acta med. Scand.* Suppl. *572* (1974).
189. Mahoney, D. H.: Intramural gastric lesion with sudden abdominal pain. *J. Amer. med. Ass. 230*, 603 (1974).
190. Teplick, J. G., Haskin, M. E.: *Roentgenologic Diagnosis*. Saunders Company, Philadelphia 1971.
191. Morley, A. P.: Obstruction of terminal small bowel and anticoagulant therapy. *Southern med. J. 63*, 342 (1970).
192. Nowotny, C., Niessner, H., Thaler, E., Lechner, K.: Sonography: A method for localization of hematomas in hemophiliacs. *Haemostasis 5*, 129 (1976).
193. Van Trotsenburg, L.: Neurological complications of haemophilia. In: Brinkhous, K. M., Hemker, H. C. (eds): *Handbook of Hemophilia*. Excerpta Medica, Amsterdam 1975.
194. Mortara, R. H., Sides, S. D., Brooks, W. H.: Removal of an intracranial glioblastoma in a hemophiliac. *Surg. Neurol. 4*, 505 (1975).
195. Mamoli, B., Sonneck, G., Lechner, K.: Intracranial and spinal haemorrhage in haemophilia. *J. Neurol. 211*, 143 (1976).

Atlas

Knee

Haemarthrosis

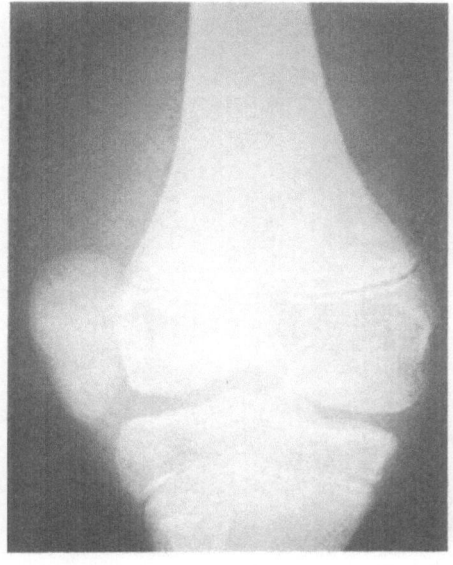

1/a

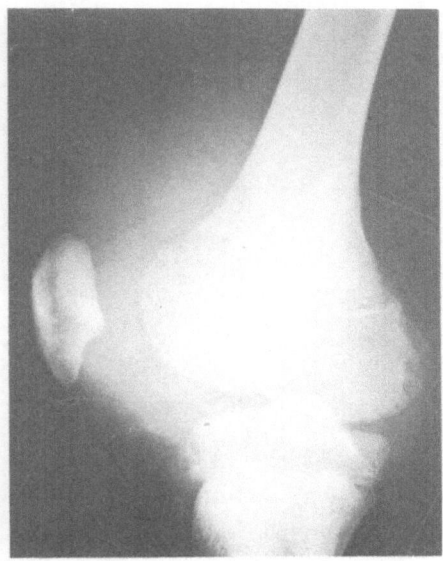

1/b

Fig. 1. T. J., 11 years, haemophilia A. Recurrent haemarthroses. Present diagnosis: acute haemarthrosis

(a, b) A–P and lateral views of the right knee. Strongly swollen periarticular soft tissue showing increased radiodensity. Lateroanterior dislocation of the patella due to intra-articular effusion

(c) A–P view of the right knee 4 years later. Irregular joint surfaces. The articular contour of the medial condyle of the femur is flattened. Note the faint subchondral sclerosis here and there. The intercondylar notch is markedly widened

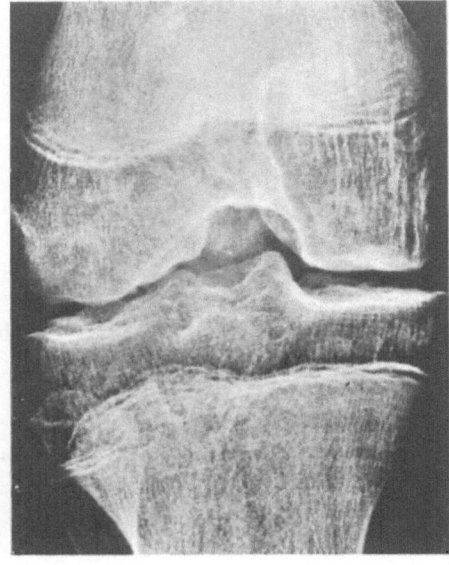

1/c

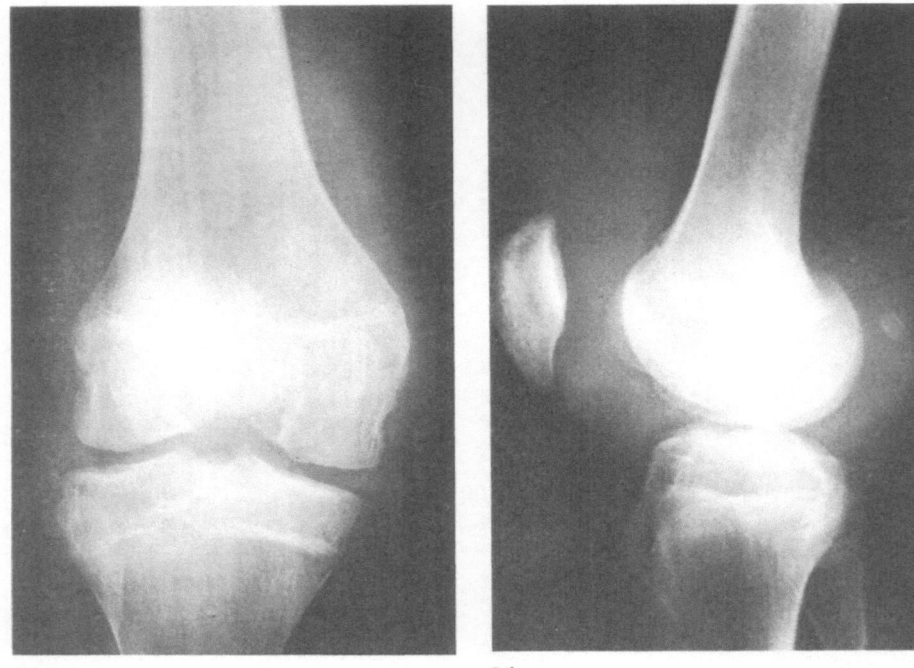

2/a   2/b

Fig. 2. K. F., 18 years, haemophilia A. Recurrent haemarthroses in the right knee

(a, b) Marked anterior dislocation of the patella. Slightly uneven articular surfaces, widened intercondylar notch

Fig. 3. U. F., 4 years, haemophilia B. Recurrent haemarthroses. Present diagnosis: acute haemarthrosis

(a, b) Comparative A–P views of the knees. The epiphyses of the right femur and tibia have lost their structure and have a balloon-like shape. The condition is due to accelerated growth and atrophy. The articular space is markedly wider than in the left knee where no haemarthrosis has occurred

(c, d) Radiographs made 4 years later. Coarse chronic atrophy on the epiphyses of the right knee, rarefaction and thickening of trabeculae. Marked resorption on the lateral edge of the tibial epiphysis: the epiphysis is narrower than the metaphysis. Uneven articular surfaces. Note Harris' lines in both knees

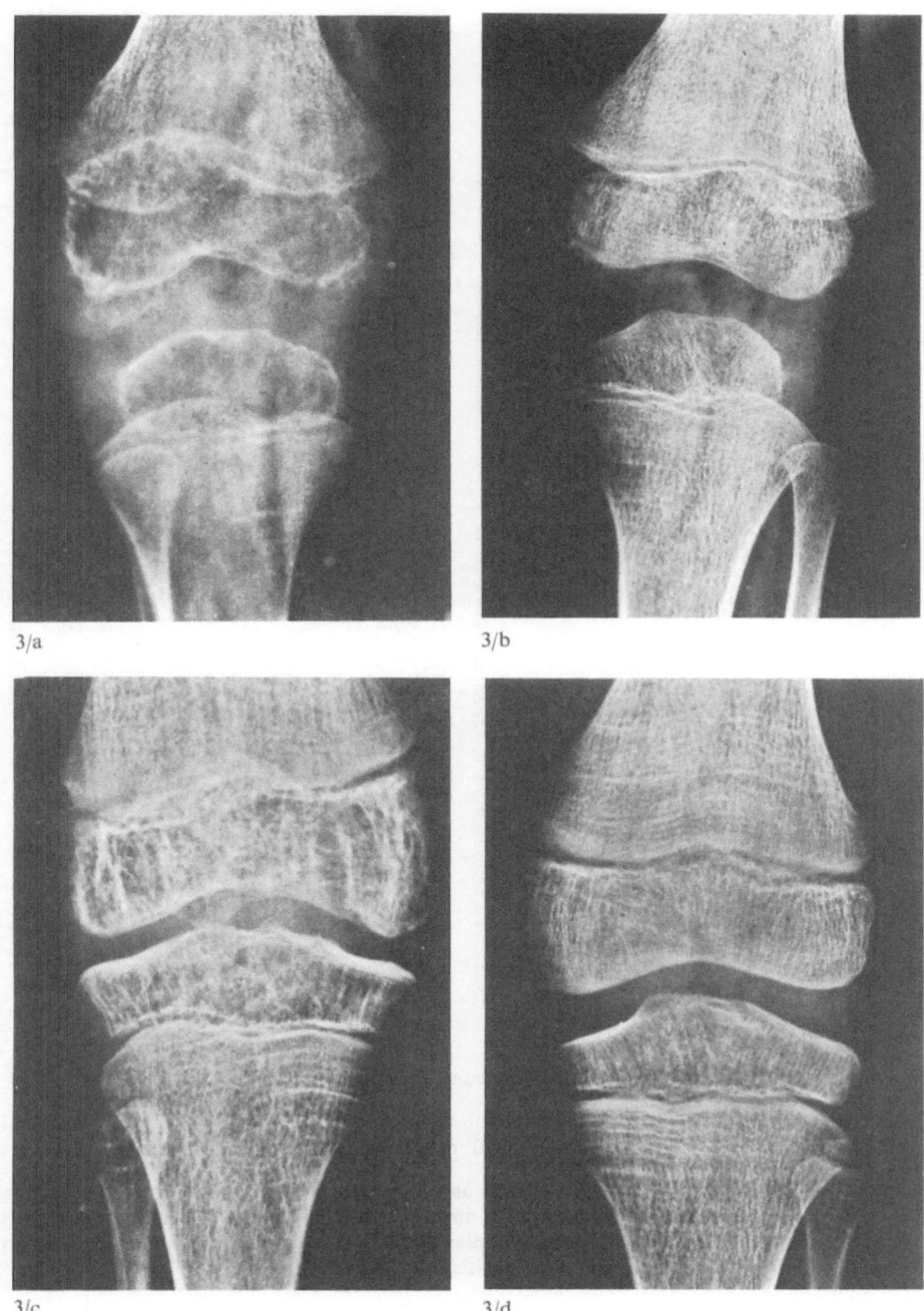

3/a

3/b

3/c

3/d

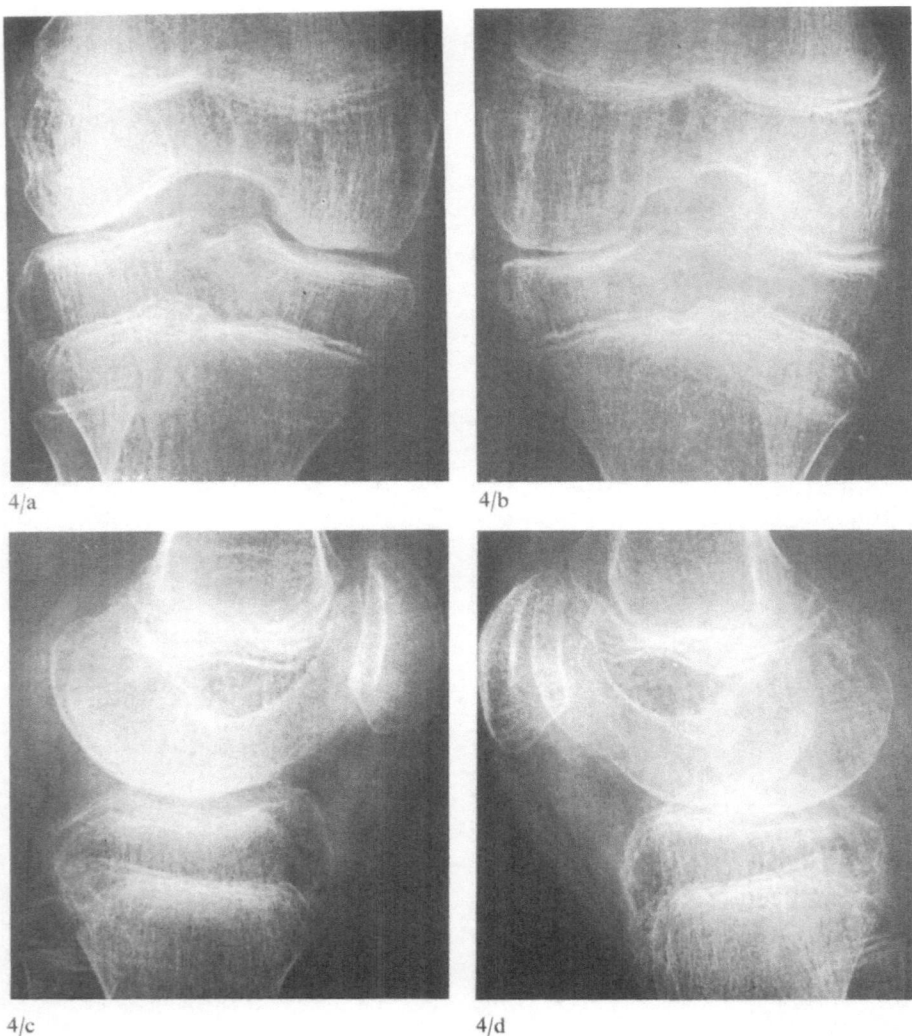

Fig. 4. D. V., 17 years, haemophilia A. Repeated episodes of bleedings in both knees

(a, b) Comparative A–P views of knees: slight, uniform chronic atrophy. Fine unevenness of the articular surfaces. Widened intercondylar notch on both sides. Narrowed joint spaces

(c, d) Comparative lateral views of knees. Squared off patella on both sides with the apices of patellae missing. Note the fine resorption directly under the epiphyseal line on the dorsal contour of the femoral condyles. Slight hypoplasia in the tibia. Signs of erosion and chondral destruction indicate transition into panarthritis

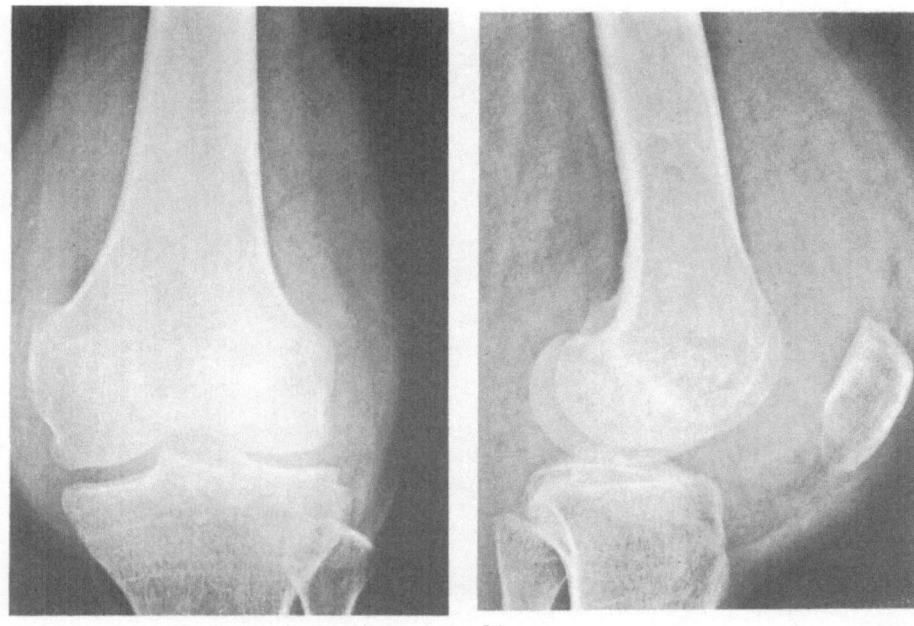

5/a   5/b

Fig. 5. M. P., 19 years, haemophilia A

(a, b) A–P and lateral views of the left knee. Marked haemarthrosis. Swollen soft tissues, patella dislocated anteriorly. Striking dilatation of the suprapatellar bursa. Note the sharp contour of resorption under the lateral edge of the articular surface of the tibia, due to hyperplasia of the synovial membrane

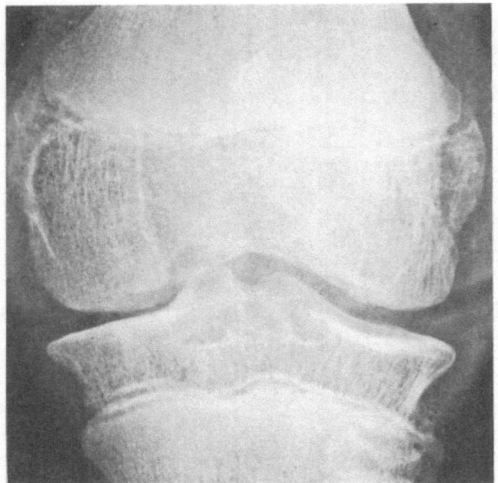

6/a

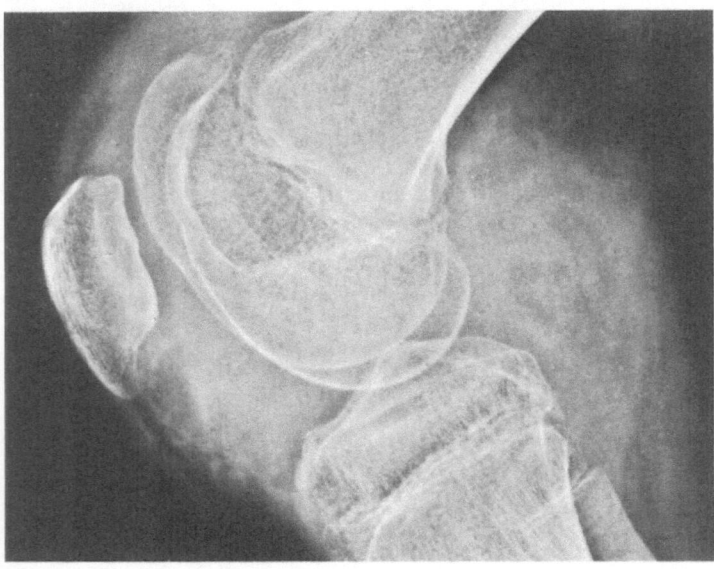

6/b

Fig. 6. B. B., 14 years, haemophilia A

(a, b) Slightly uneven articular surfaces, narrowed joint space. Marked marginal resorption on both sides of the tibial epiphysis. The contours of the femoral condyles are sharp, indicating extreme atrophy

Panarthritis

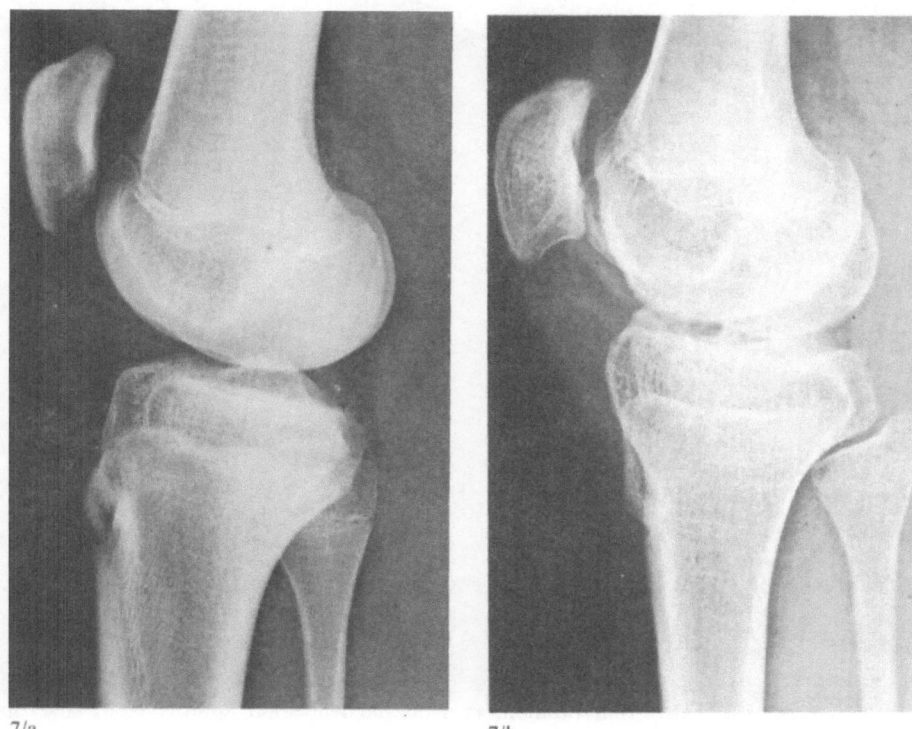

7/a   7/b

Fig. 7. H. Gy., 15 years, haemophilia A

(a, b) Lateral view of both knees. The right knee is intact. Left knee: squared off patella. Narrowed articular space, uneven articular surfaces. On the left side advanced fusion of the epiphyses due to recurrent haemarthroses. The anterior contours of the femoral condyles are flattened. The diaphysis of the tibia is hypoplastic as compared with its normally developed epiphyses. Squared off patella has only developed in the arthropathic joint, supporting the view that this alteration is not congenital, but the result of a local process

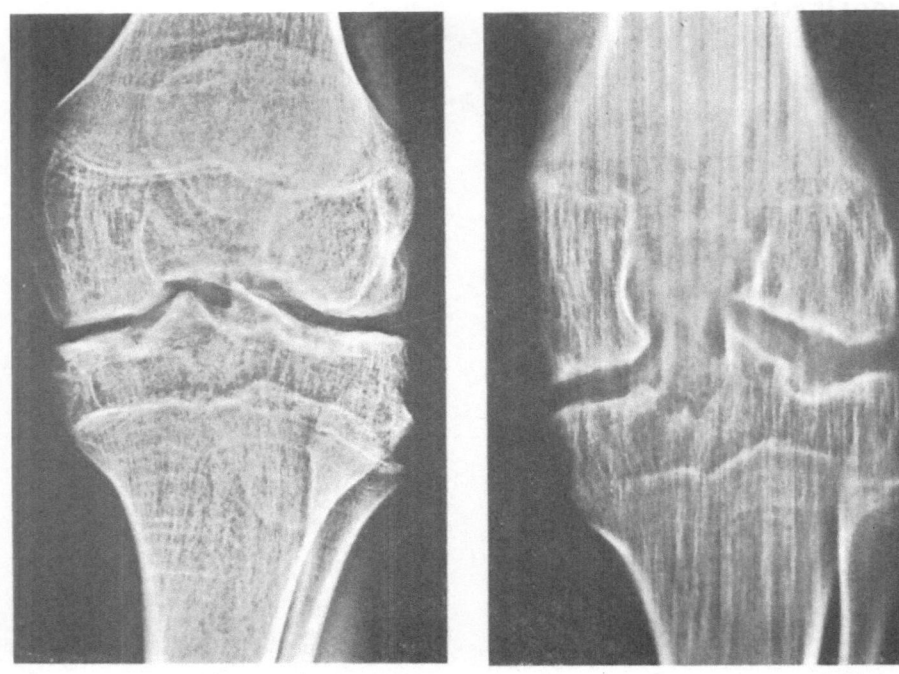

7/c   7/d

Fig. 7

(c, d) Left knee. A–P view. Frontal tomogram. Note the depression, approximately fingertip deep, on the lateral part of the tibial articular surface. The opposing joint surface of the femur is markedly flattened. The articular surfaces are uneven. The lateral intercondylar tubercle is pointed. Note exostosis on the internal edge of the lateral condyle of the femur (internal osteophyte). Fine rarefactions under the articular surfaces

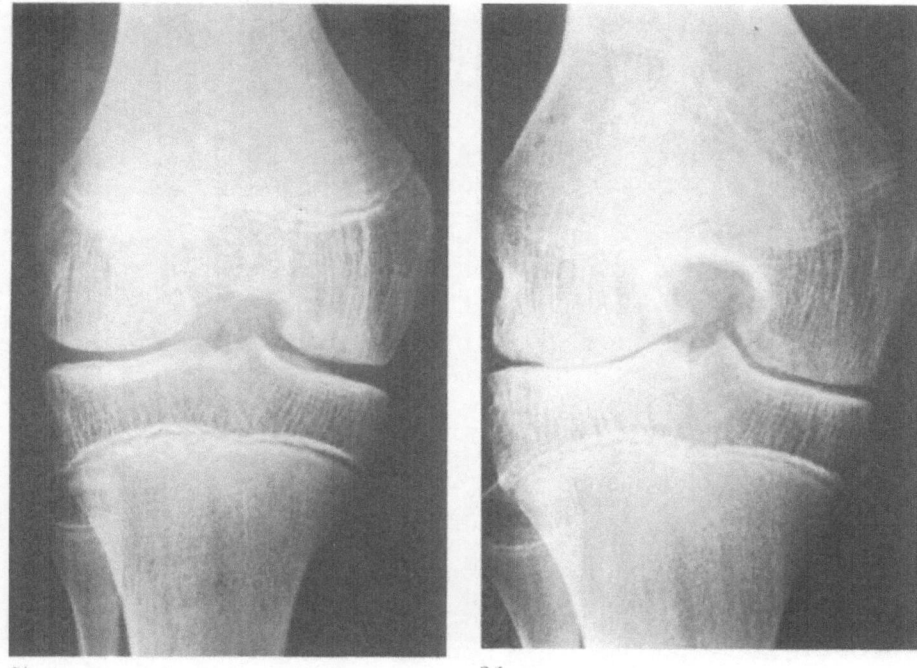

8/a   8/b

Fig. 8. K. A., 14 years, haemophilia A

(a) A–P view of the right knee. The joint space is slightly narrowed, the intercondylar notch slightly widened

(b) The same joint 2 years later. Markedly narrowed joint space, the articular surfaces are uneven, the intercondylar notch is markedly widened, the intercondylar tubercles are deformed. The progression of the process during the two years is striking

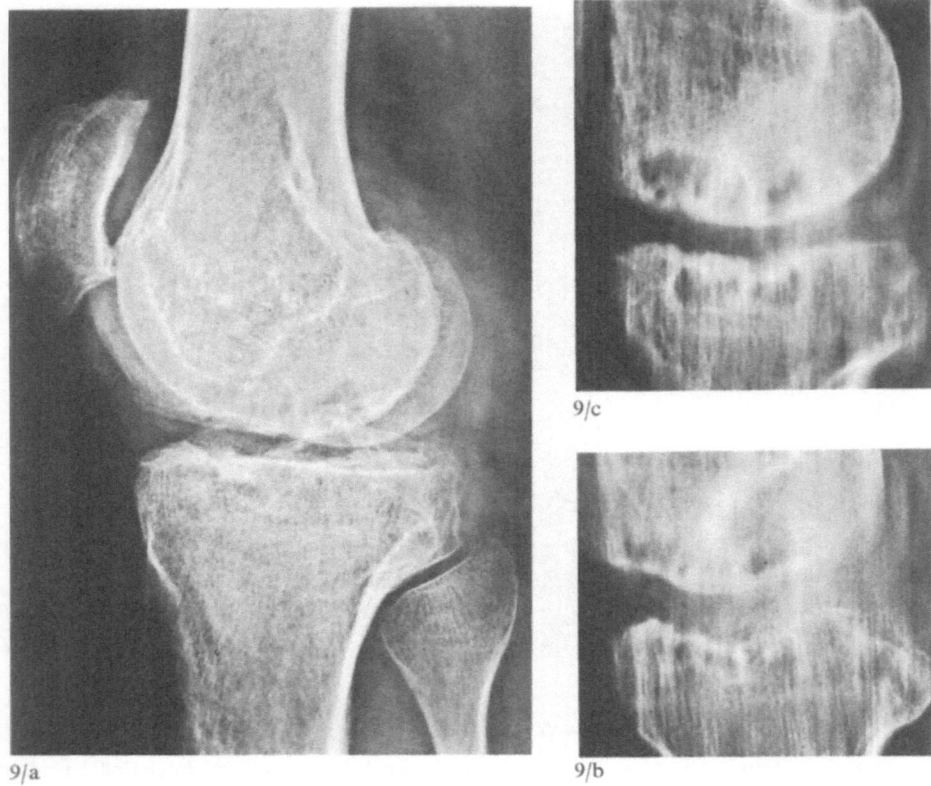

9/c

9/a

9/b

Fig. 9. Sz. J., 24 years, haemophilia A

(a–c) Uneven articular surfaces. Sagittal tomograms reveal the pea- to bean-sized subchondral rarefactions, above which the joint surface is fragmented and has in some parts broken in

Fig. 11. S. Gy., 29 years, haemophilia B

(a, b) In the lateral condyle of the tibia a plum-sized cyst, with a sclerotic border, communicating with the articular space. Uneven articular surfaces, deep intercondylar notch

Fig. 10. L. J., 23 years, haemophilia A

Plumstone-sized oval cyst in the medial condyle of the tibia. The medial half of the joint space is markedly narrowed. The intercondylar notch is widened, its lateral ridge bears a thorn-like prominence (internal exostosis). Note that the subchondral process has taken place at the site where the cartilage has been destroyed

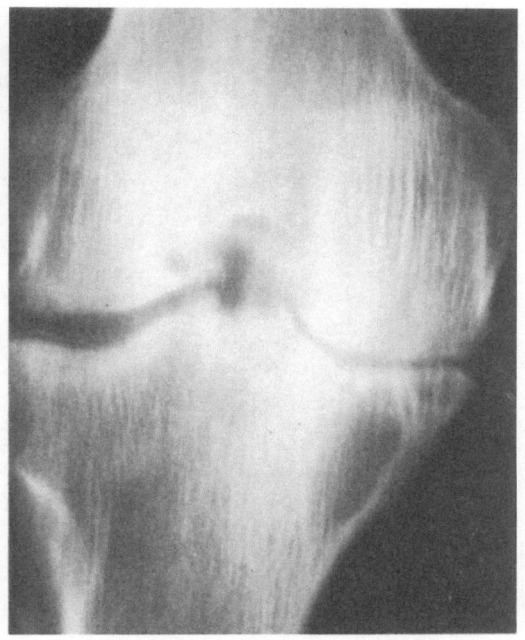

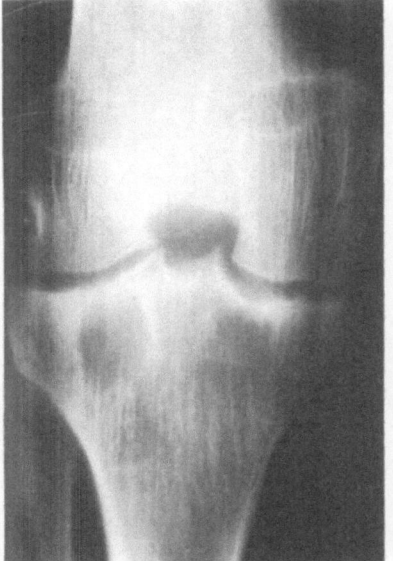

11/a

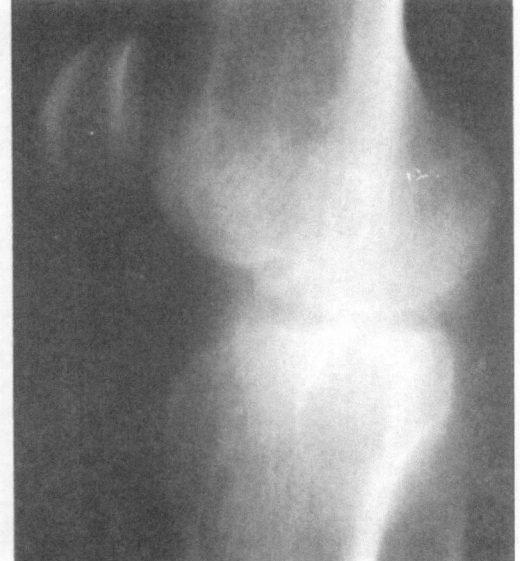

11/b

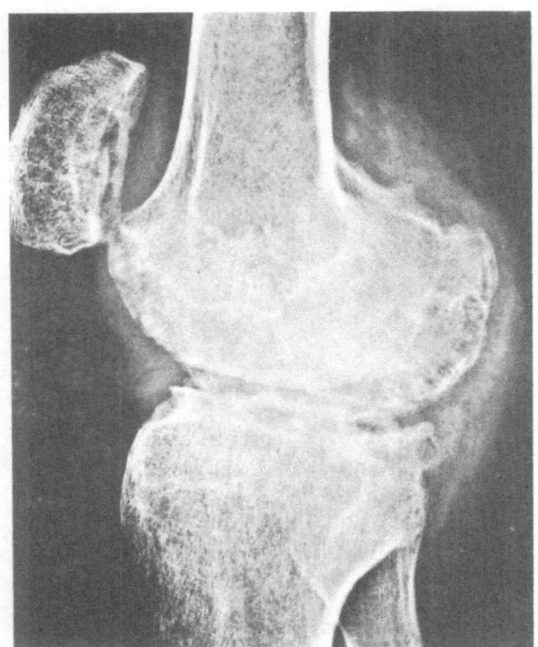

12/a

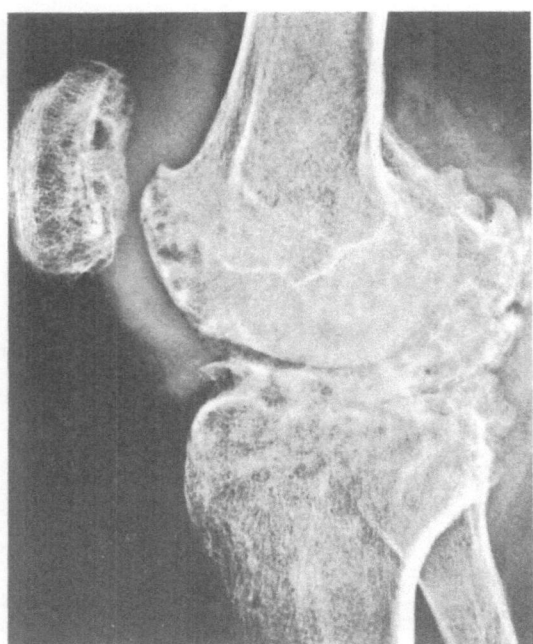

12/b

Fig. 12. T. Cs., haemophilia A

(a) Lateral view of right knee at 24 years of age. Squared off patella, narrowed joint space, uneven contours. String-like series of lentil-sized subchondral cysts along the wavy articular surfaces

(b) Three years later. The alterations have advanced considerably. Markedly uneven articular surfaces, many of the subchondral cysts communicate with the joint space. The anterior pseudoosteophyte of the tibia has also grown

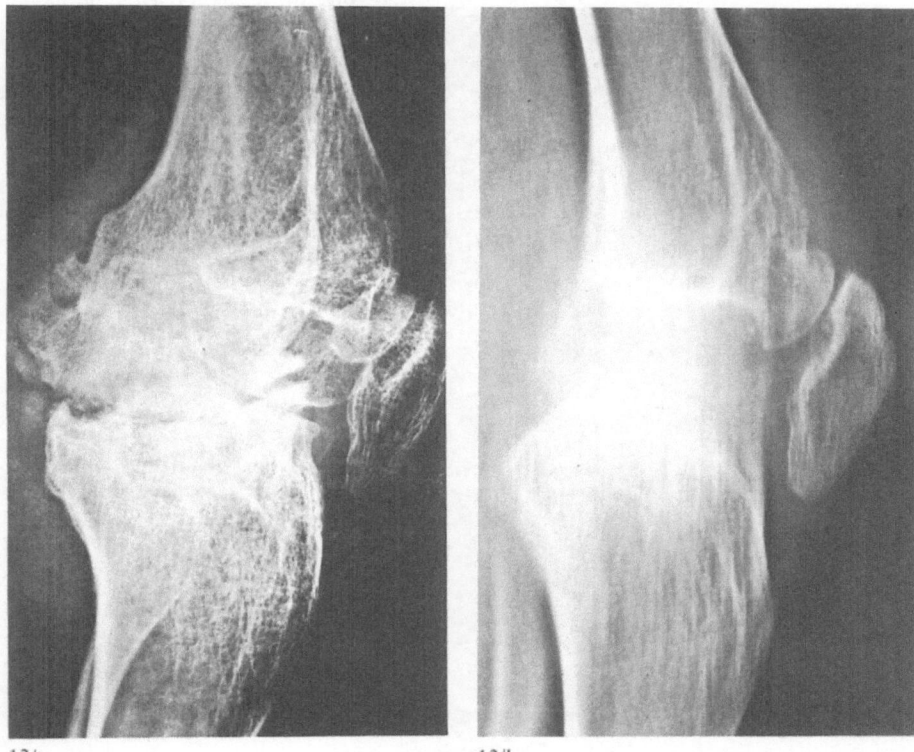

13/a 13/b

Fig. 13. B. F., 25 years, haemophilia A

(a, b) Lateral view reveals serious arthropathy. The irregularity of the posterior femoral contour is striking. Anterior osteophytes of both femur and tibia. The tomogram displays the medial depth of the joint: the deep intercondylar notch has undermined the anterior articular surface of the femur, forming an almost independent plumstone-sized process. The articular surface of the patella is pitted

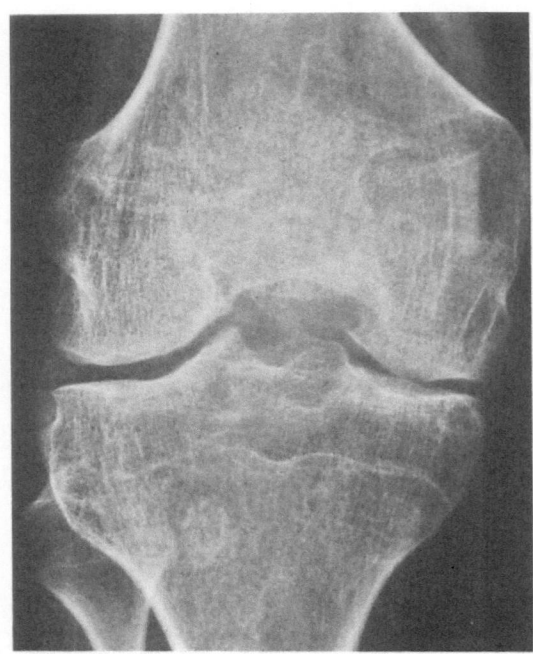

Fig. 14. R. B., 14 years, haemophilia A

(a, b) Right side: slight alterations. Left side: marked narrowing of the articular space, marked resorption on the medial edge of the tibia

14/a

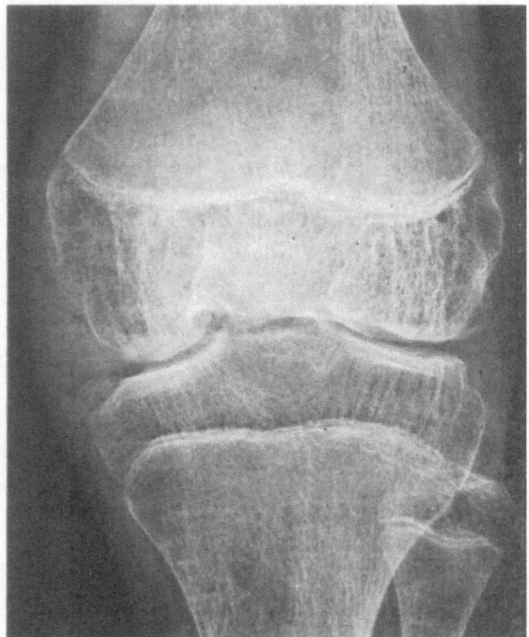

14/b

(c, d) Follow-up radiograph. Advanced alterations 5 years later

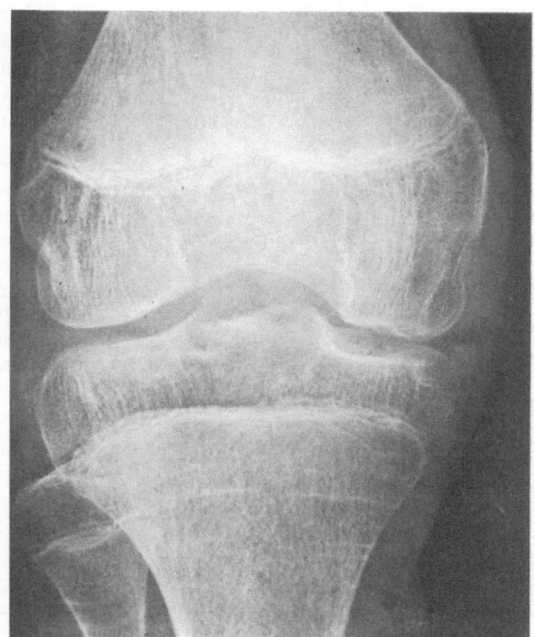

14/c

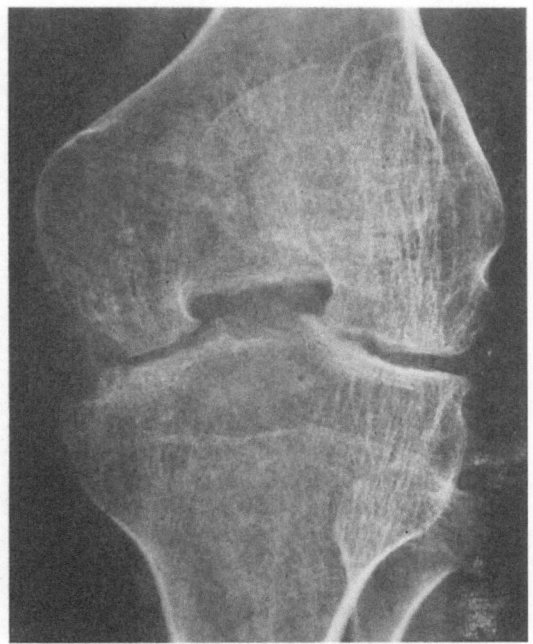

14/d

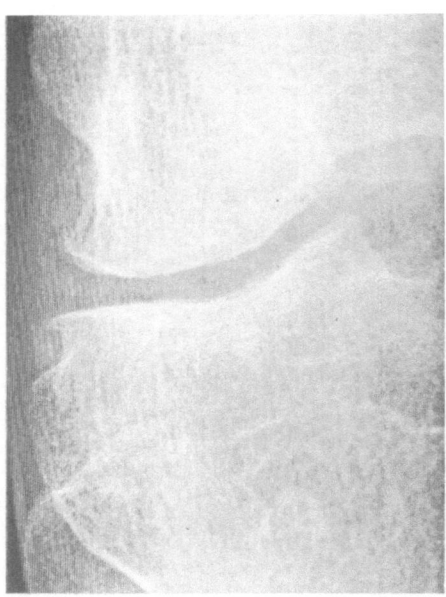

14/e

Fig. 14

(e) Magnified picture of the lateral edge of the right knee. Note the pseudoosteophyte on the edge of the tibia which results from the undermined articular surface

(f) Direct X-ray magnification of the left knee. Coarse resorption on the medial condyles of both the femur and the tibia, resulting in a considerable shortening of the articular surfaces, particularly that of the lateral condyle of the femur, which is about half in length of the opposing surface. Uneven articular surfaces, deep intercondylar notch. Typical structure of chronic atrophy

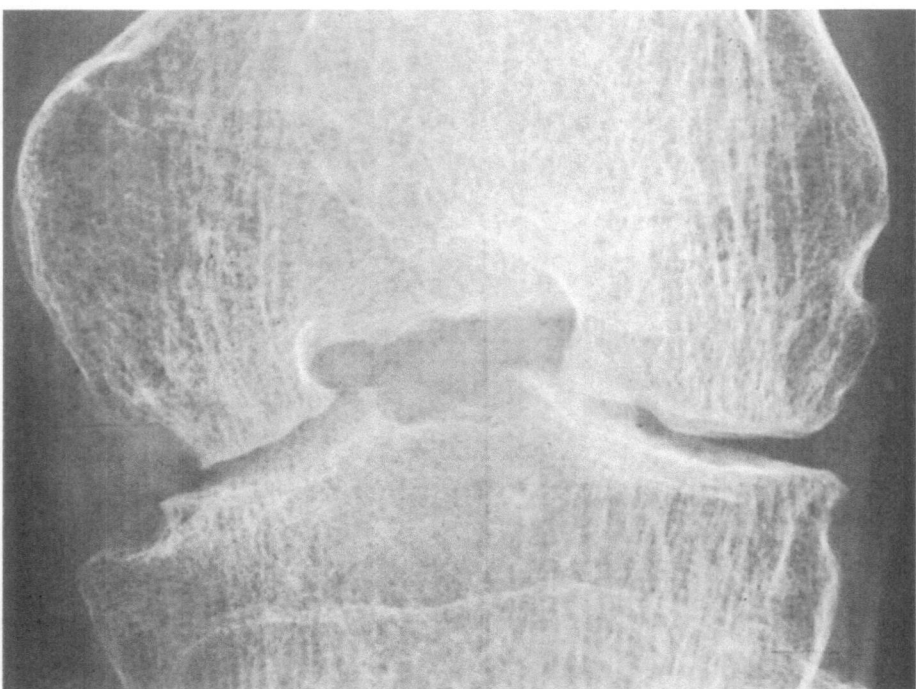

14/f

(g) Left knee, lateral view. The condyles of the femur are markedly flattened anteriorly, the entire epiphysis is hypoplastic. As a result of ventral resorption, the articular surface of the tibia is strikingly shortened. Squared off patella

(h) Direct X-ray magnification of 14/g

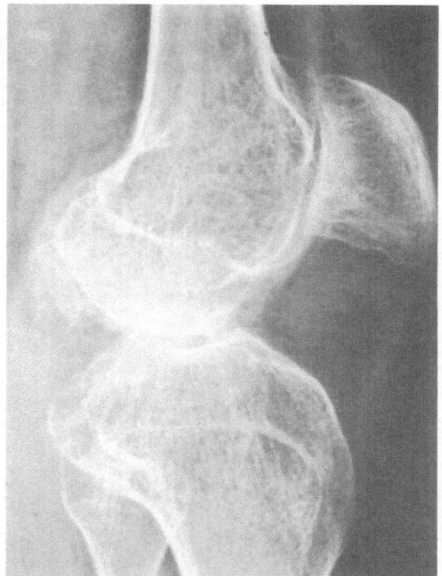

14/g

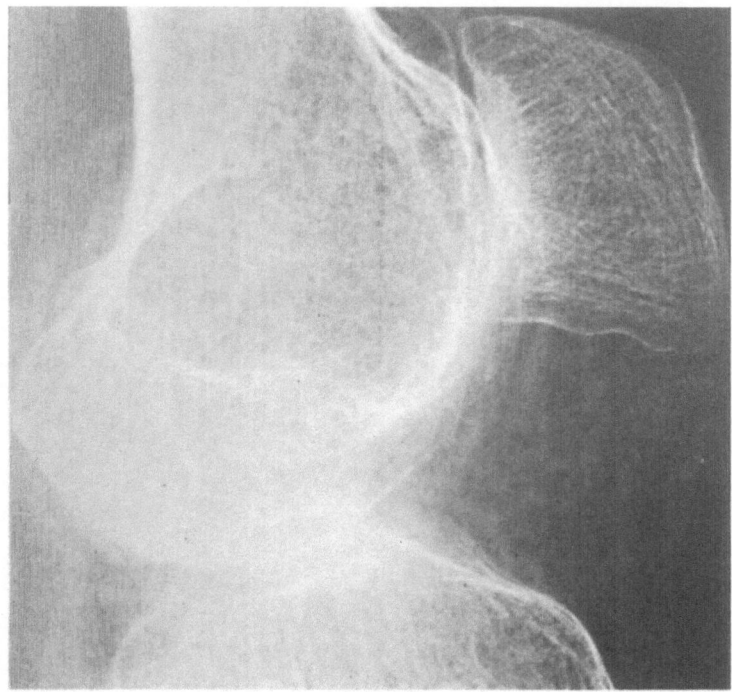

14/h

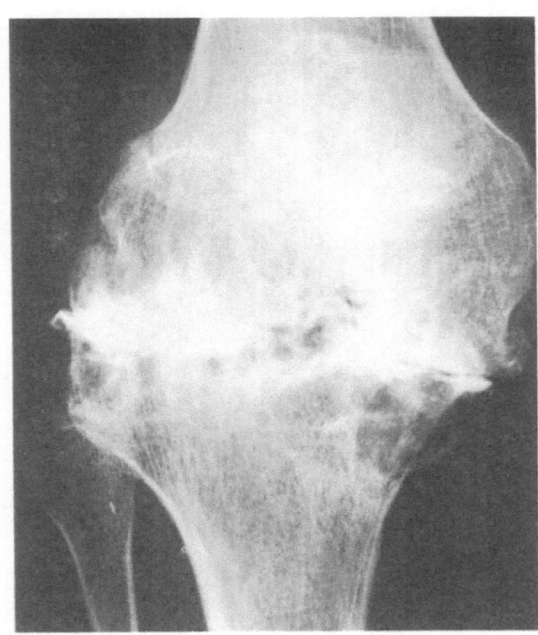

15/a

Fig. 15. M. J., 70 years, haemophilia A

(a, b) A–P and lateral views of the right knee. Joint space almost totally obliterated, extensive coarse sclerosis, many cysts

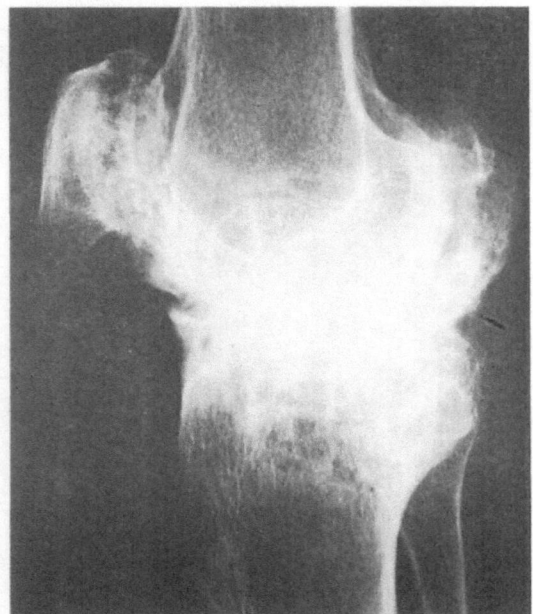

15/b

Fig. 16. T. A. K., 60 years, haemophilia A

(a, b) Frontal and sagittal tomograms of the right knee. Besides the typical alterations, the ventral subluxation of the tibia is striking. Marked subchondral sclerosis, fragmented articular surfaces, many cysts

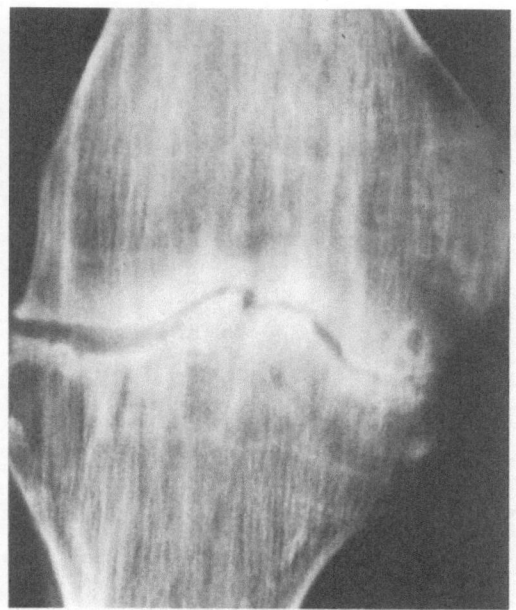

16/a

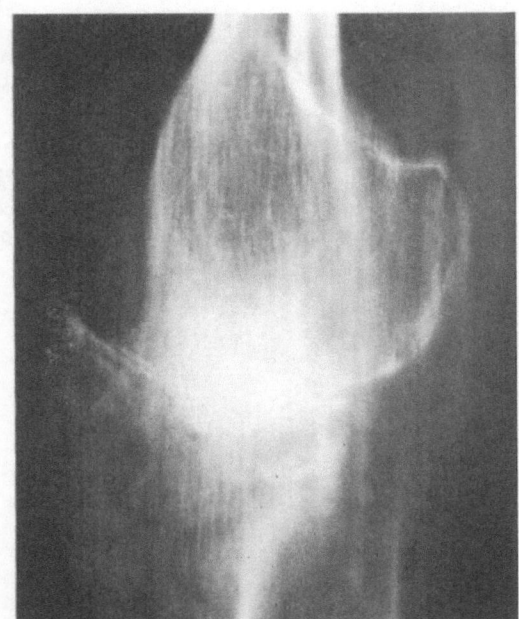

16/b

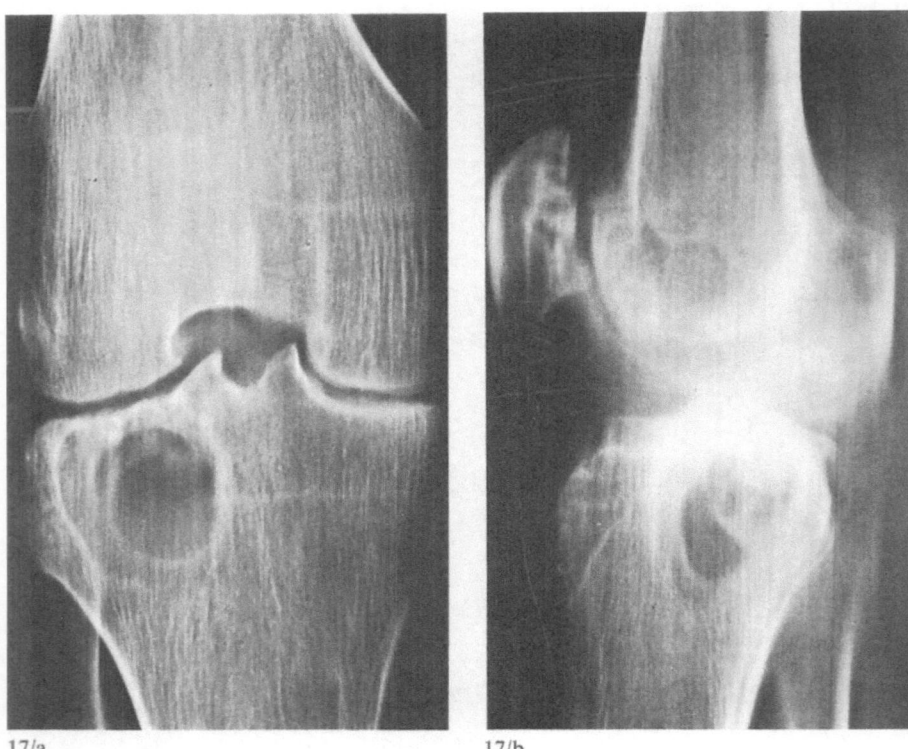

17/a   17/b

Fig. 17. G. J., 23 years, haemophilia A

(a, b) Tomograms of the right knee, A–P and lateral view. In the lateral condyle of the tibia a green-nut-sized cyst. Above it, the articular surface is pitted. The joint surface of the medial condyle is intact. Many subchondral cysts in the patella

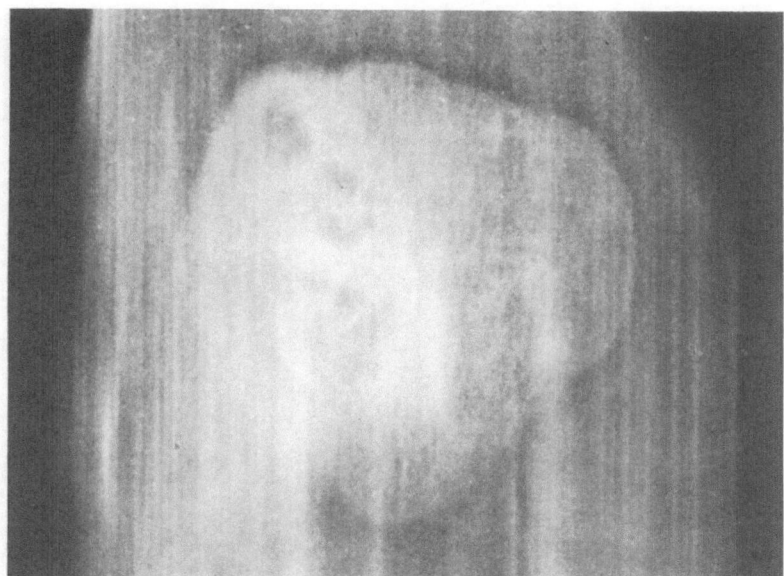

17/c

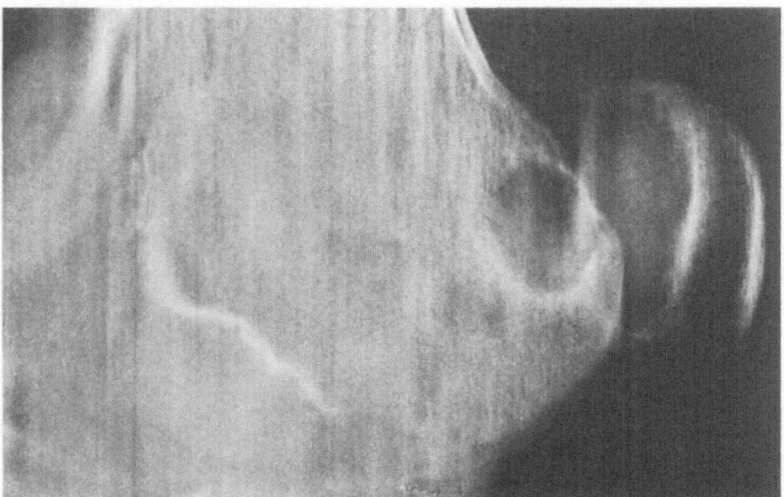

17/d

(c) Frontal tomogram of the patella. Note the small cysts in the external upper quadrant

(d) Oblique tomogram. Cherry-sized cyst under the patellar joint surface of the femur. Above it, the contour is uneven

73

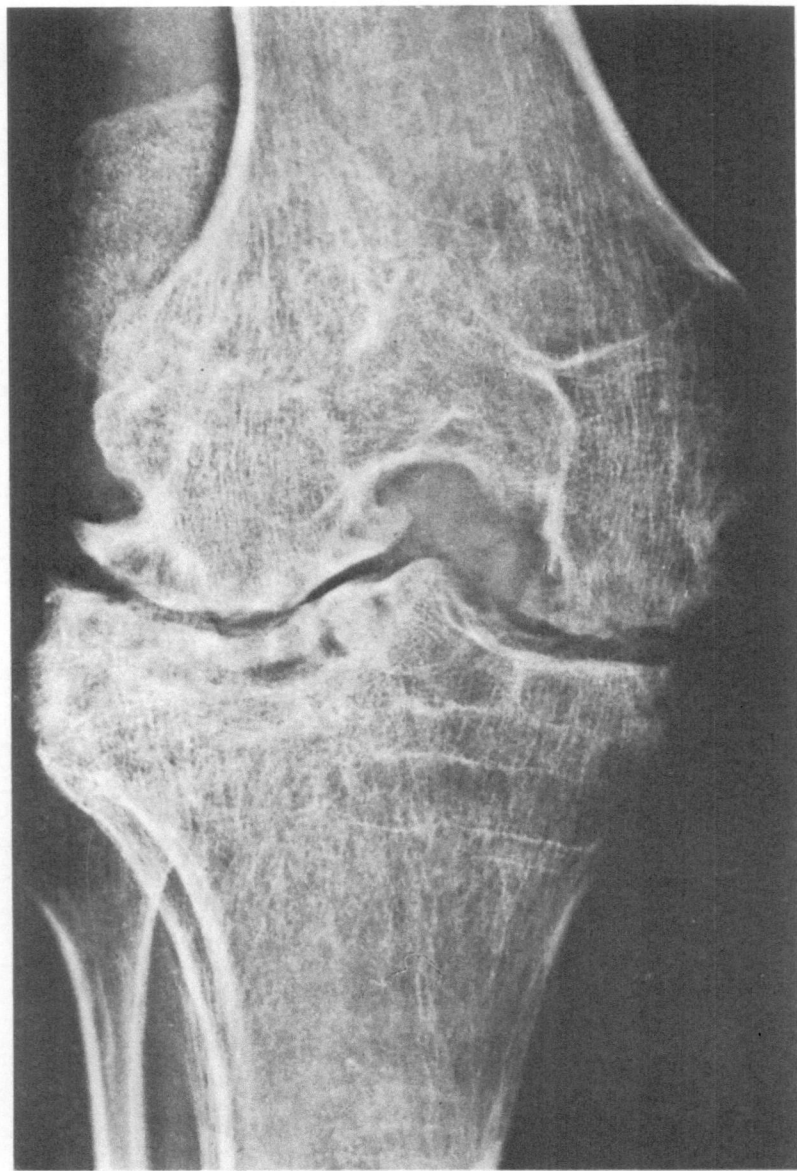

18/a

Fig. 18. S. J., 25 years, haemophilia A

(a, b) Right knee. Frontal projection. The lateral condyle of the femur is mushroom-shaped as a result of resorption. Irregular joint surfaces, many subchondral cysts

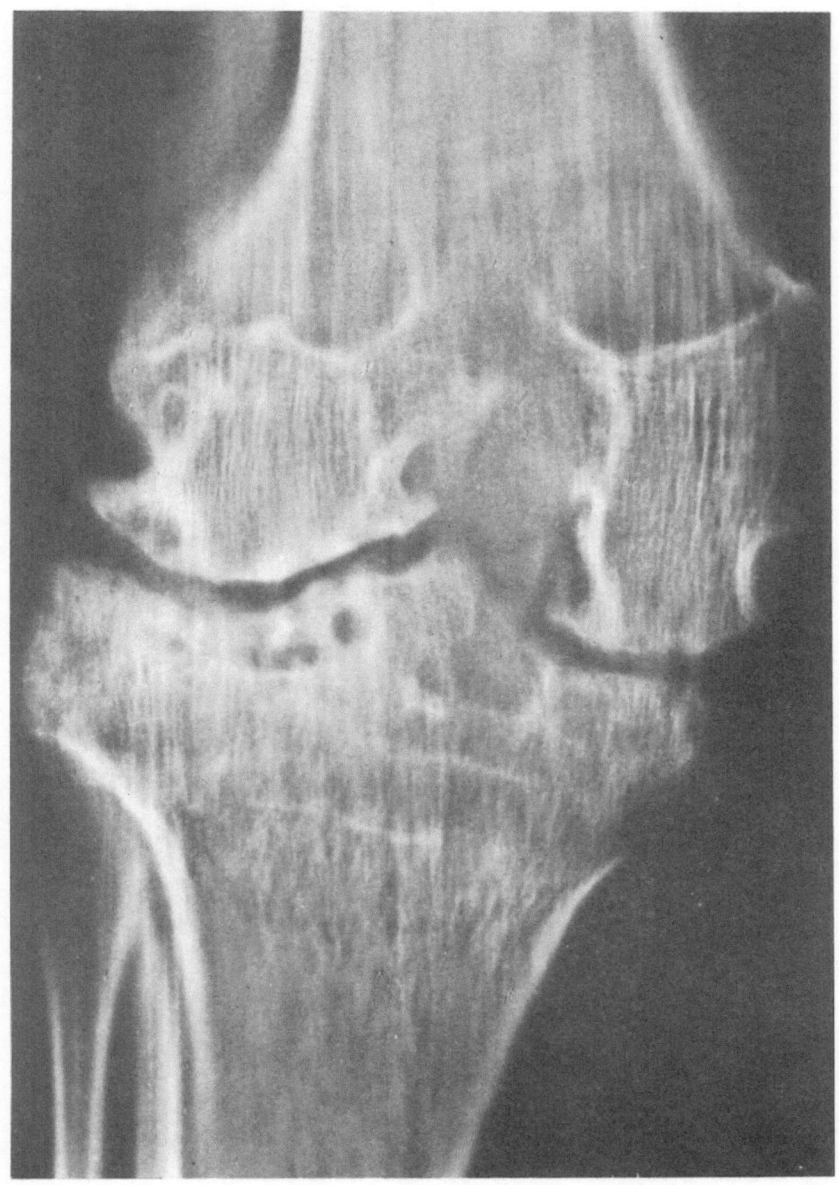

18/b

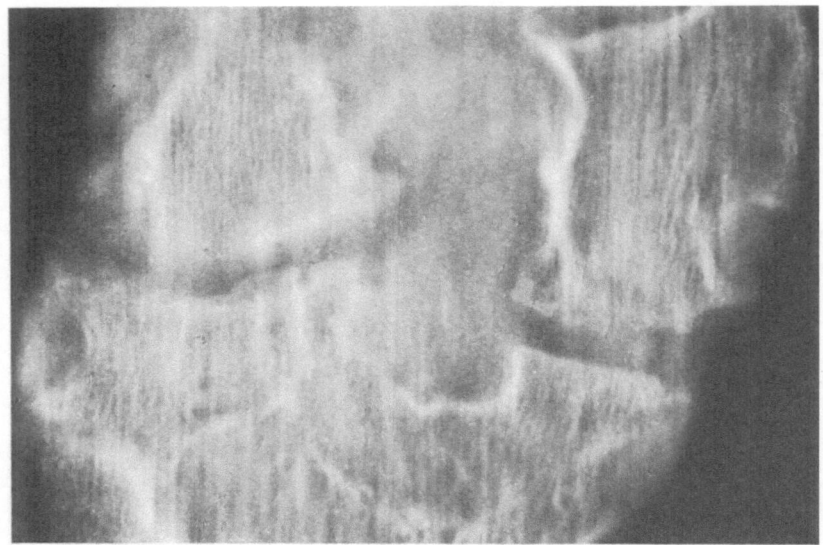

18/c

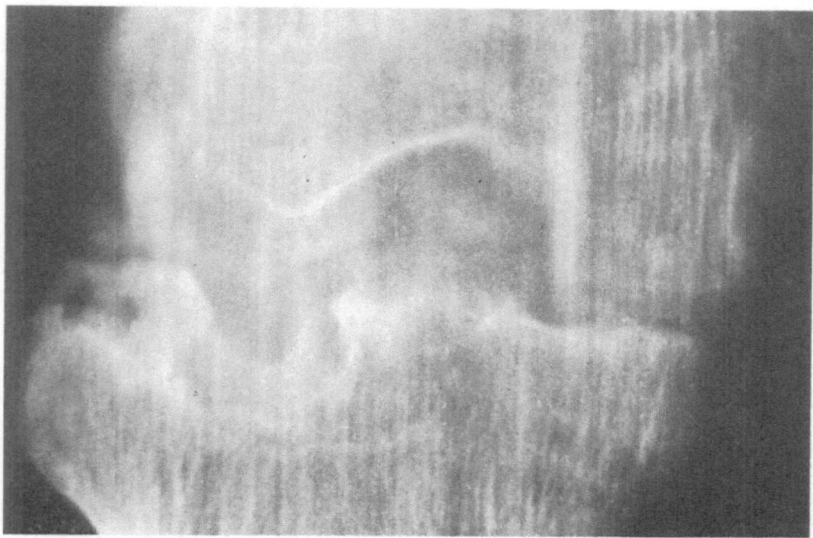

18/d

Fig. 18

(c, d) Impressions of different depths with sclerotic borders in the articular surface of the tibia, which are, in fact, cysts widely communicating with the joint space

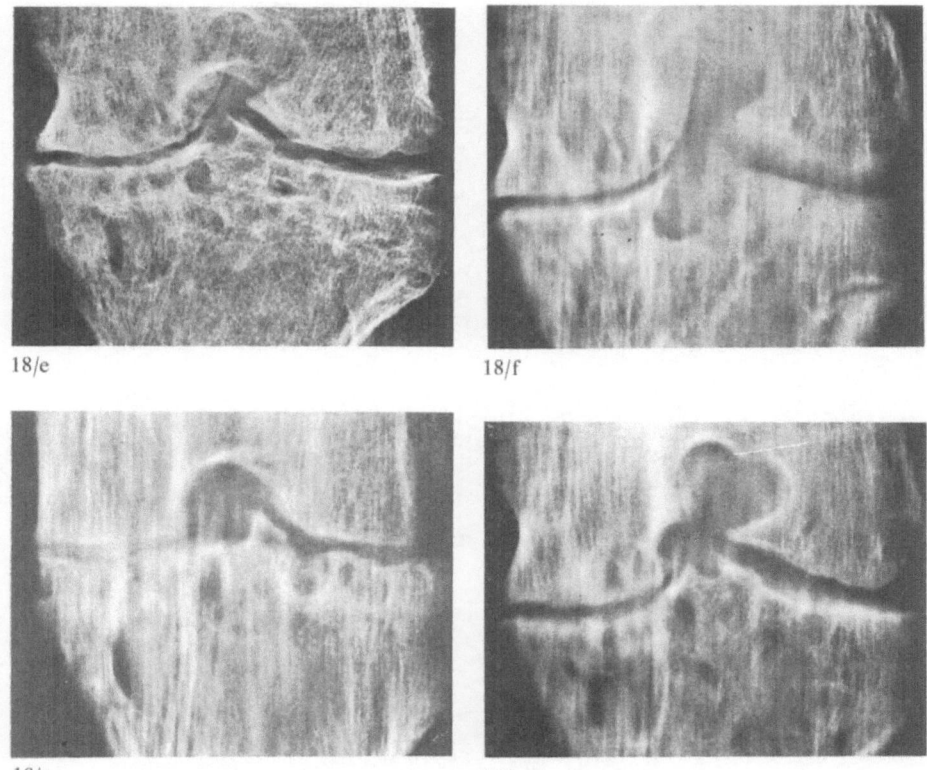

18/e

18/f

18/g

18/h

(e–h) Left knee. Numerous subchondral cysts of lentil- to cherry size, some of them communicating with the articular space

(f) Tomogram. A giant internal pseudoosteophyte on the medial condyle of the tibia

(g) Tomogram. Beside the lateral intercondylar tubercle, there is a peanut-sized cyst communicating widely with the joint space

(h) Tomogram. Flattening of the lateral condyle of the femur and a typical internal pseudoosteophyte forming the distal-lateral edge of the deepened intercondylar notch

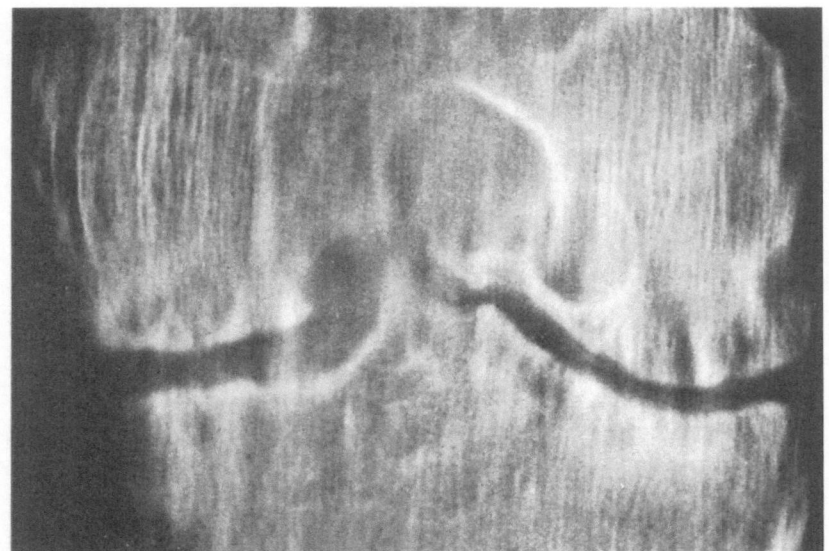

19/a

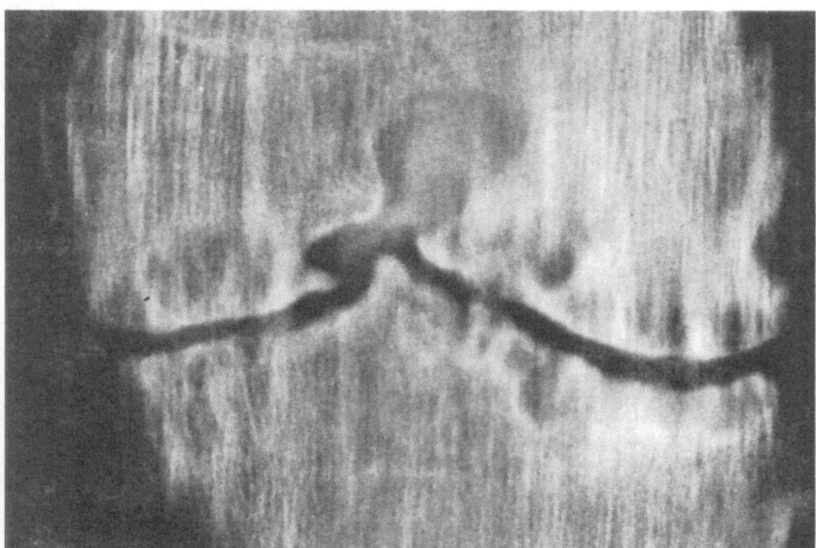

19/b

Fig. 19. K. J., 20 years, haemophilia A

(a, b) Numerous cysts. Fragmented joint surfaces. Narrow articular space. An internal pseudoosteophyte on the medial condyle of the femur

Regression

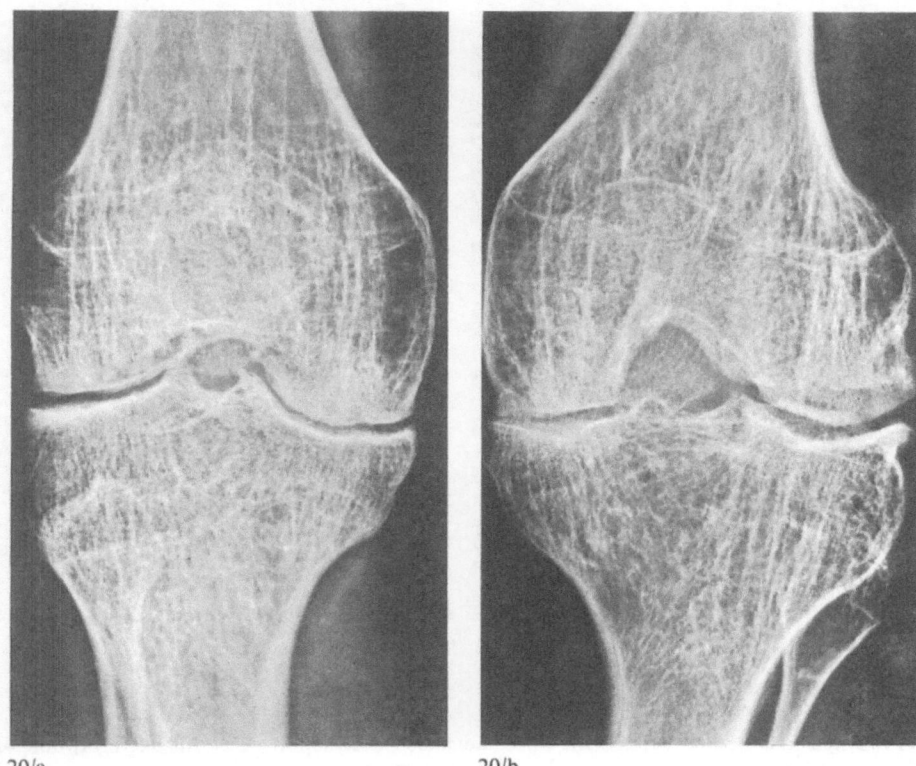

20/a   20/b

Fig. 20. H. S., 30 years, haemophilia B

(a, b) After numerous recurrent haemarthroses a quiescent condition in both knees. Markedly narrowed articular spaces, irregular joint surfaces, deepened intercondylar notch. Bone structure corresponding to marked chronic atrophy. The trabeculae are rarefied and thickened

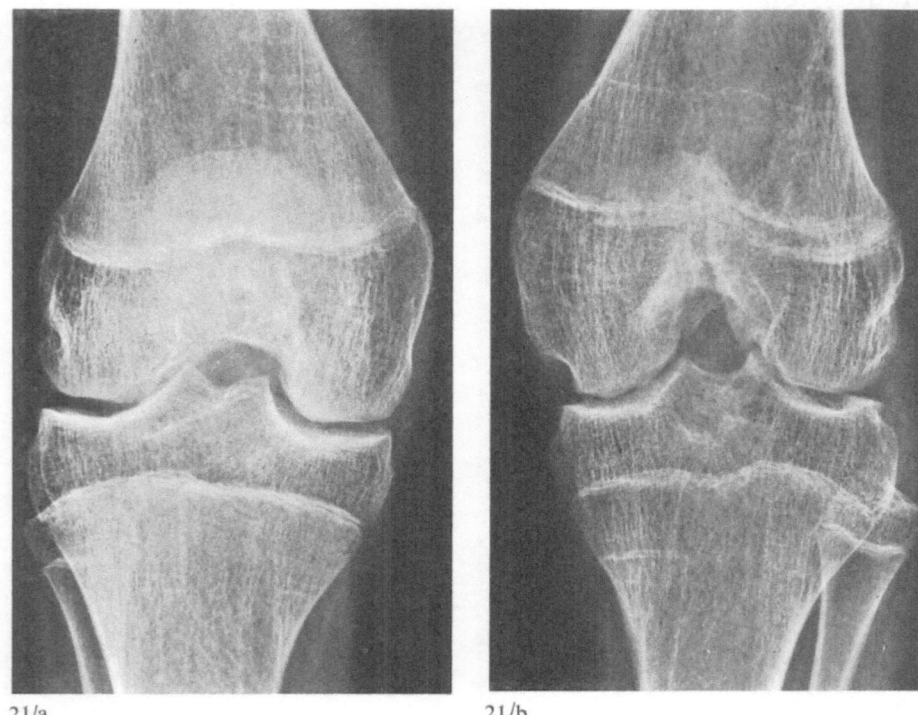

21/a   21/b

Fig. 21. P. L., 14 years, haemophilia A

(a, b) Right knee: panarthritis. Left knee: advanced destruction of cartilage, resorption of chondral edges, and a marked atrophy indicating regression

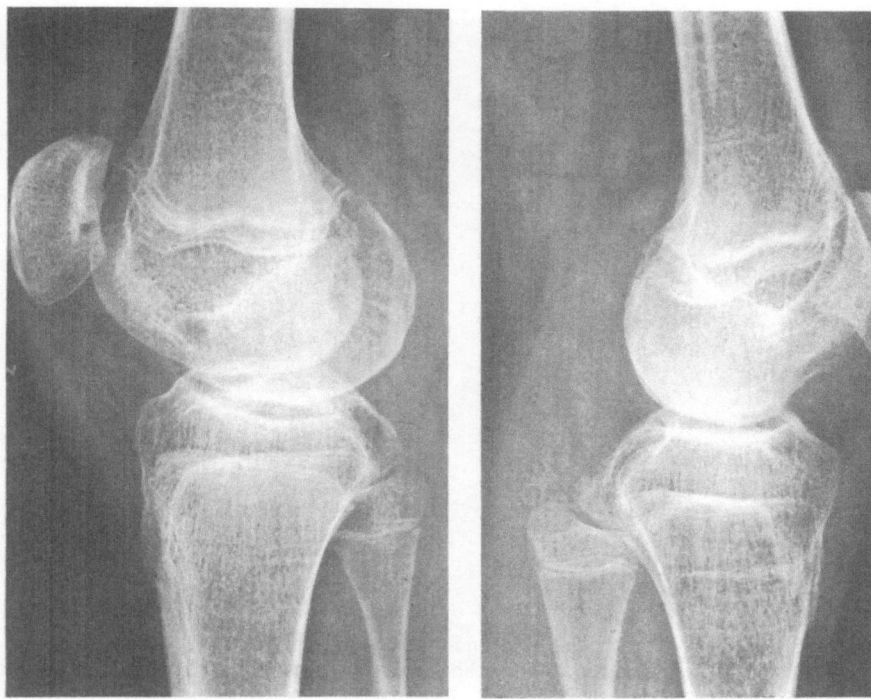

21/c   21/d

(c, d) The same joints in lateral view. Left knee: underdeveloped bone-ends, hypoplastic metadiaphysis of the tibia, squared off patella. This case demonstrates that some patients reach the stage of regression at an early age

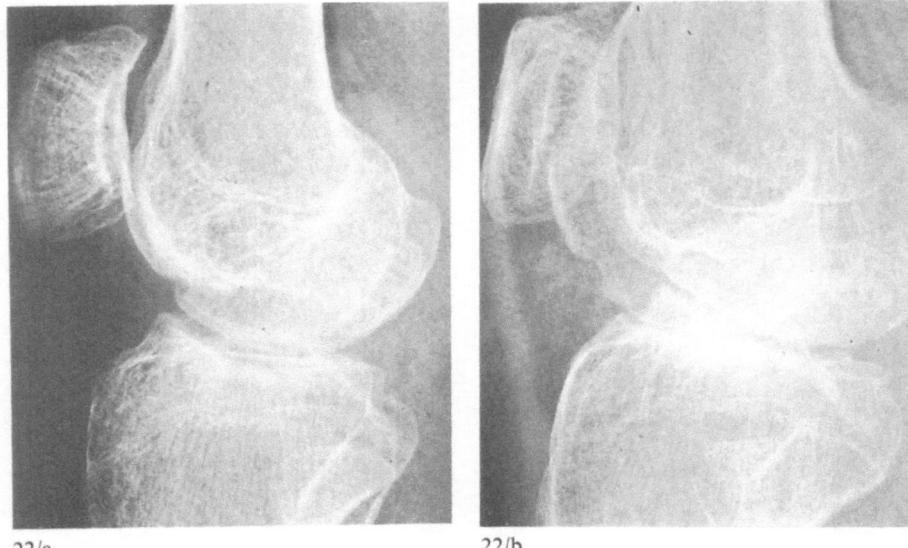

22/a   22/b

Fig. 22. R. N., 22 years, haemophilia A

(a) Marked regression. The crude lytic and sclerotic alterations have been replaced by more regular structures. The condyles of the femur are hypoplastic. Squared off patella

(b) The same knee 16 years later. Degenerative sequelae have become more marked, otherwise no basic change is visible. The fundamental course can be considered terminated at 22 years of age. In the subsequent 16 years no specific progression took place

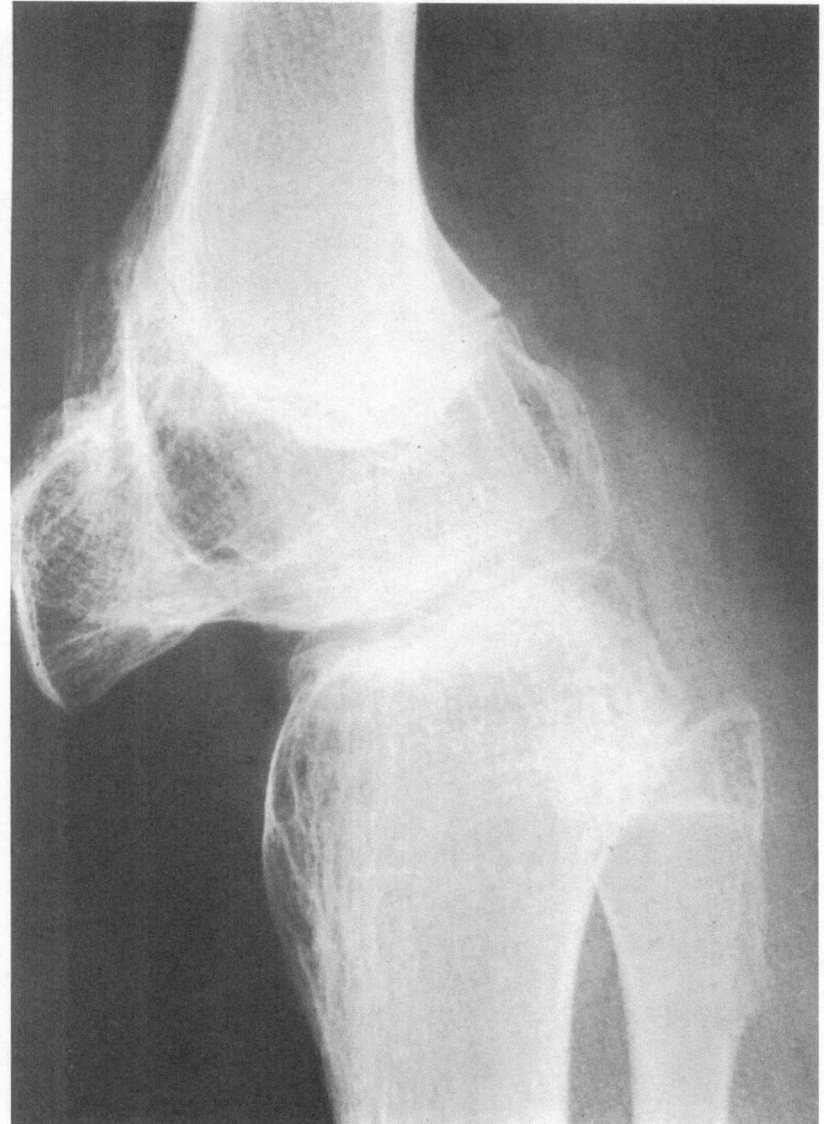

Fig. 23. P. J., 17 years, haemophilia A

Lateral view of the right knee. The direction of the articular space is anterodistal, the bone-ends are underdeveloped. Osseous ankylosis between the femur and the squared off patella. The pathological process has terminated by the age of 17 years

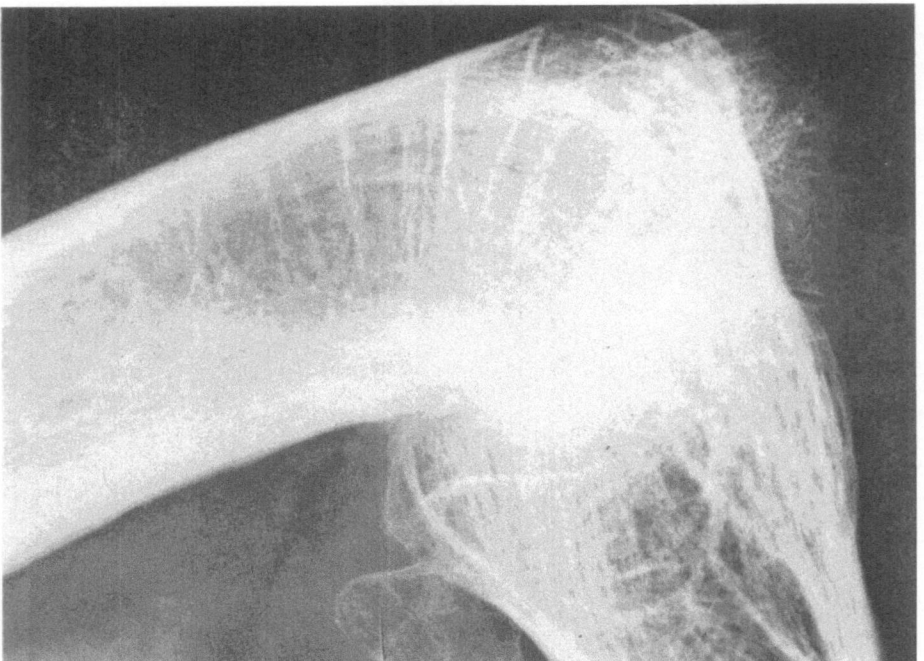

24/a

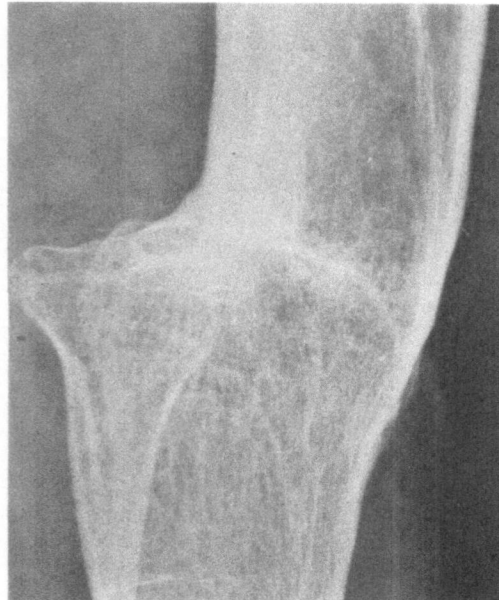

Fig. 24. R. N., 22 years, haemophilia A

(a) Total osseous ankylosis in the knee, 90° contracture. With progression of chronic atrophy the structure of the trabeculae has become adapted to the new statical conditions: the thickened trabeculae at the distal end of the femur are perpendicular to the longitudinal axis of the bone

(b) Postosteotomic condition

24/b

84

Ankle

Haemarthrosis

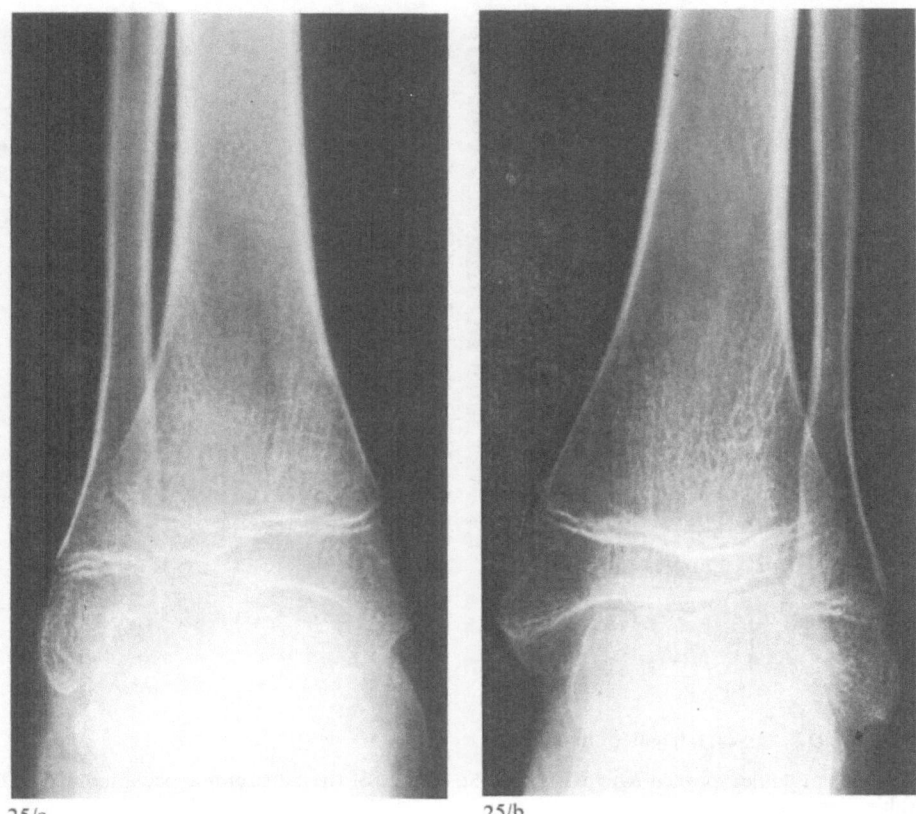

25/a   25/b

Fig. 25. D. V., 17 years, haemophilia A

(a, b) The distal epiphysis of the tibia displays a characteristic alteration on both sides: the epiphyses are considerably narrowed in lateral direction, and they have a pointed lateral edge. The trochlea of the talus is also irregular in shape: it slopes upwards in the lateral direction. Hence, the articular space tends upwards obliquely from the medial-distal to the lateral-proximal end

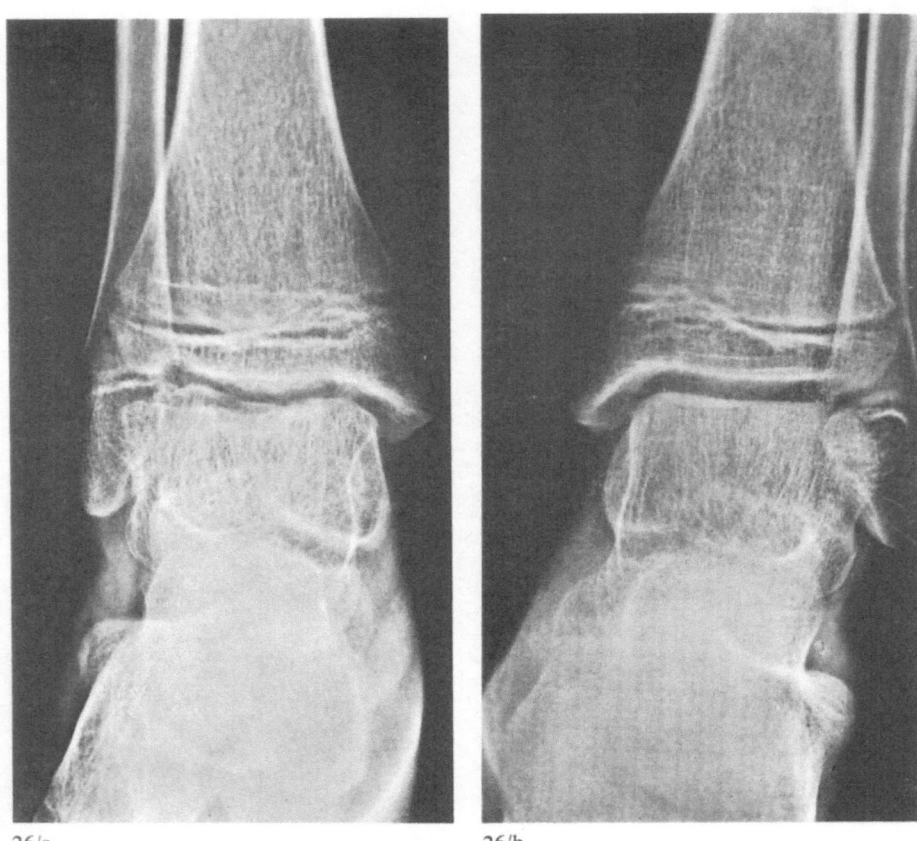

26/a 26/b

Fig. 26. P. O., 11 years, haemophilia A

(a, b) Right ankle: marked irregularity on the surface of the talocrural articulation. The left ankle is intact (c, d) Lateral view: fine erosion on the anterior aspect of the right trochlea of the talus. Slight atrophy. No cysts

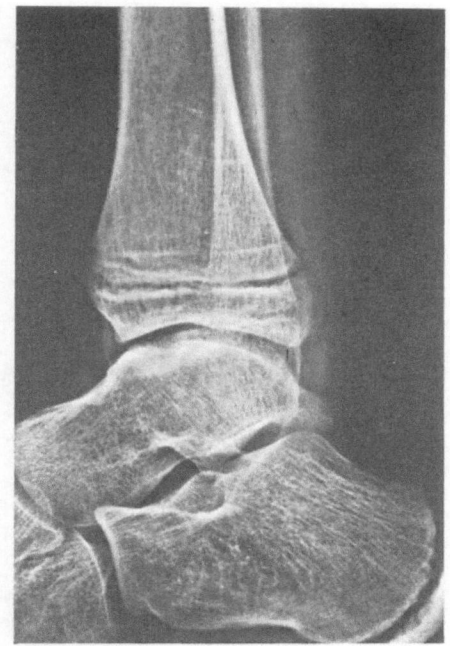

26/c

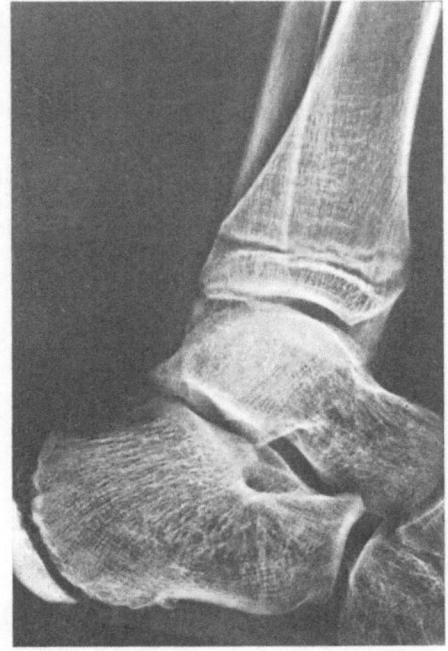

26/d

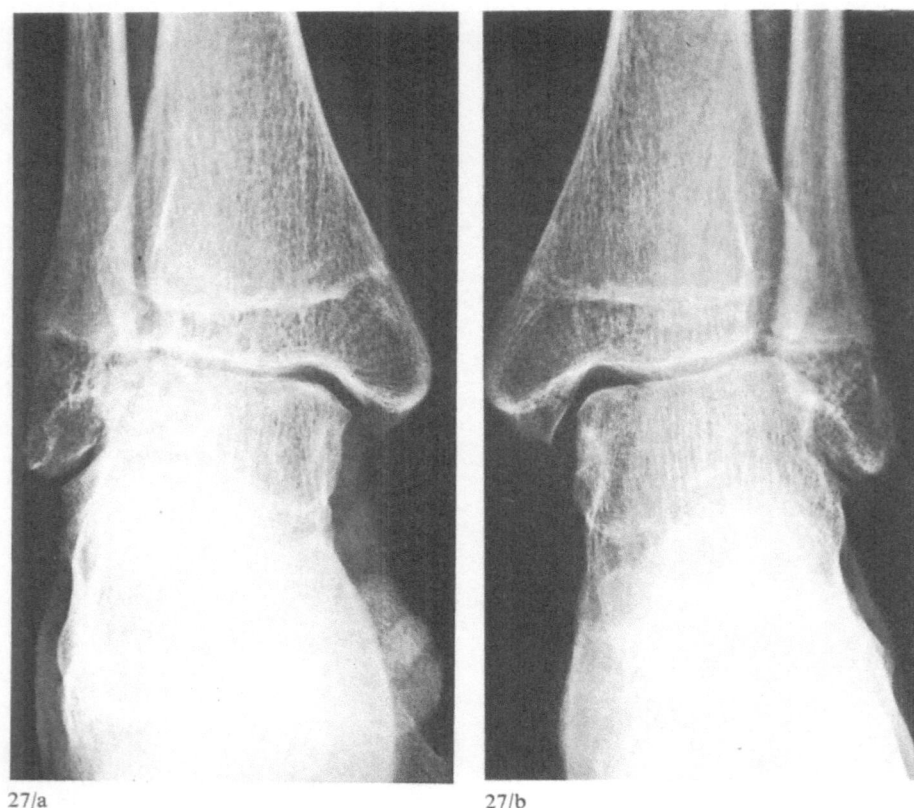

27/a   27/b

Fig. 27. B. I., 18 years, haemophilia A

(a, b) Right ankle: advanced state. Left ankle: slight alterations. Note the irregular shape of the distal epiphysis of the tibia. On the right side, where the articular surface is markedly uneven, rarefactions are visible in the trochlea of the talus

Fig. 28. S. Gy., 29 years, haemophilia A

(a–c) Cysts under the uneven talar surface. The tomograms display large cysts in the distal epiphysis of the tibia and in the talus. The anterior cyst in the tibia communicates with the joint space, the highest point of the trochlea of the talus is pitted

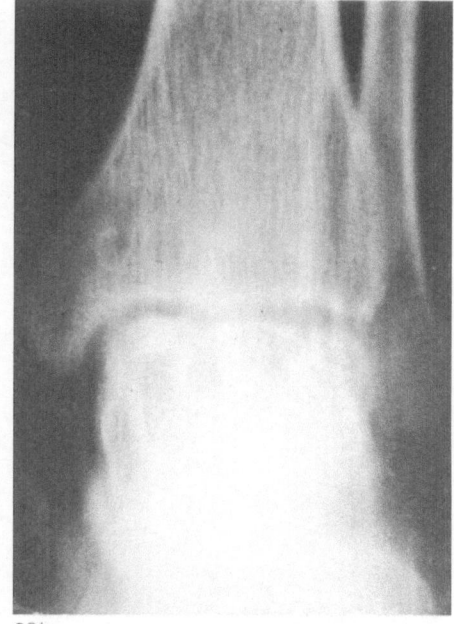

28/a

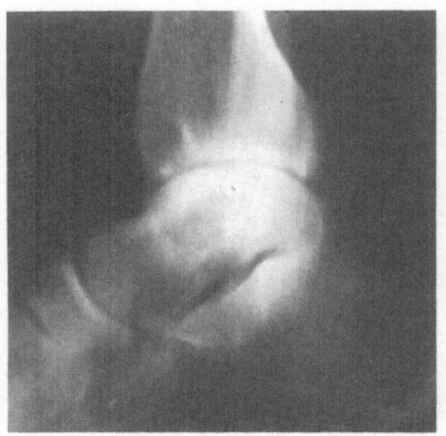

28/b

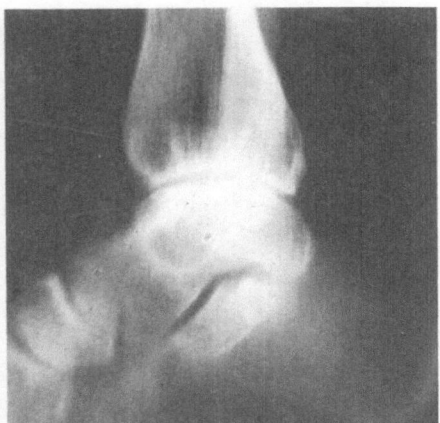

28/c

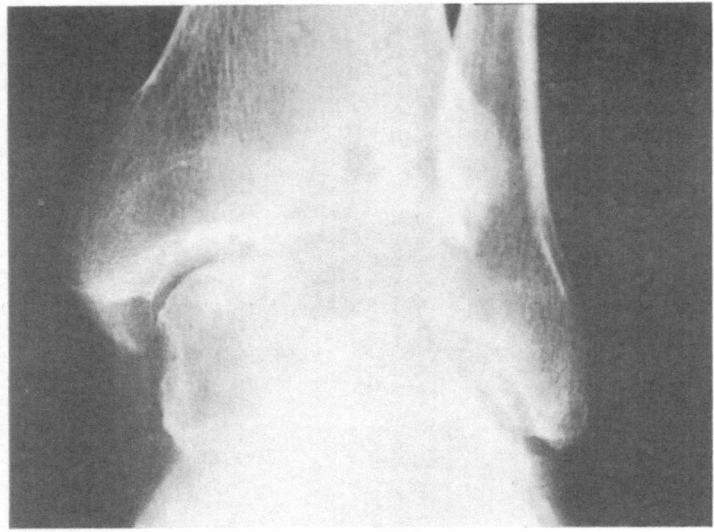

29/a

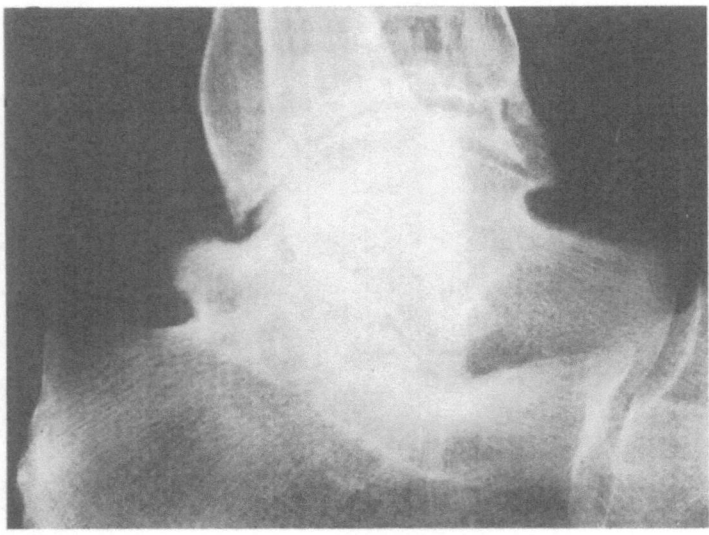

29/b

Fig. 29. M. J., 70 years, haemophilia A

(a, b) Subchondral cysts in the sclerotic substance of the tibia are striking. The contour of the talus is undermined at the ventral edge of the articular surface

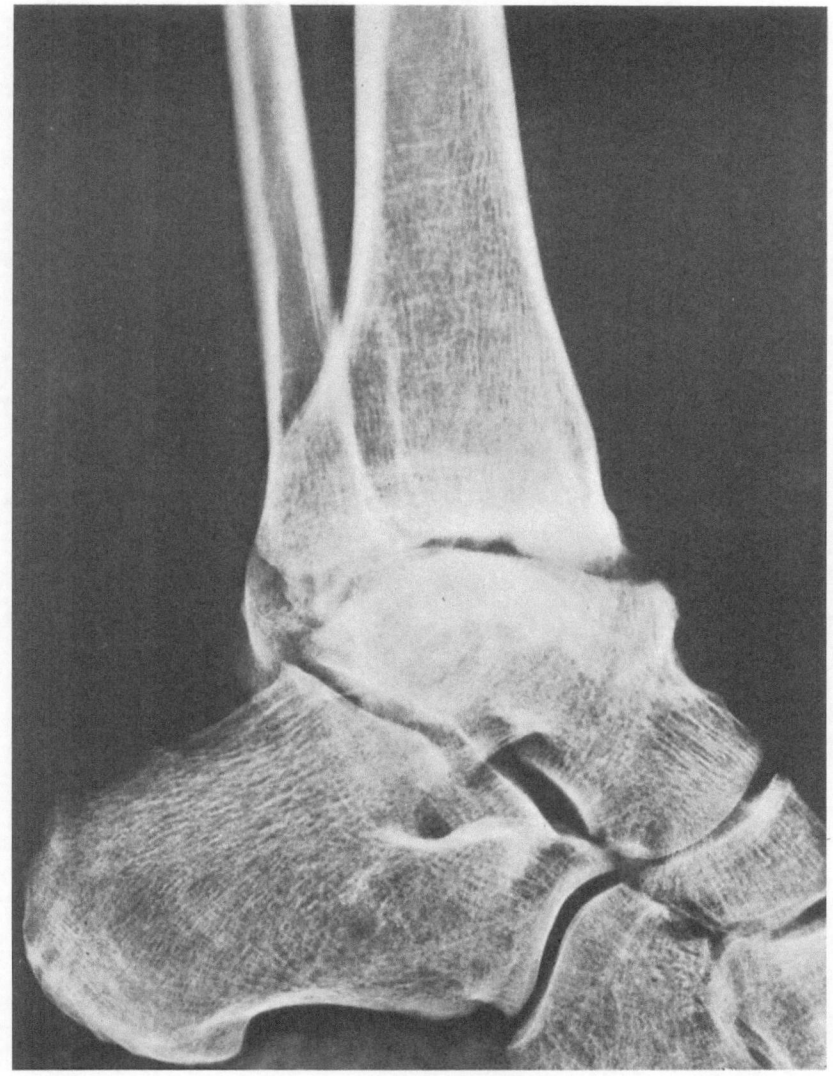

Fig. 30. N. Gy., 39 years, haemophilia A

Severe deformity and sclerosis remind of tabetic arthropathy, the intertarsal joints are intact

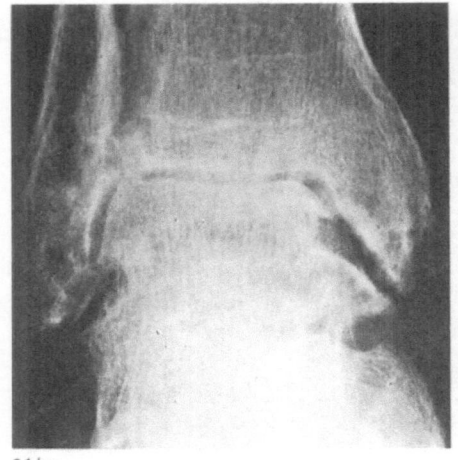

31/a

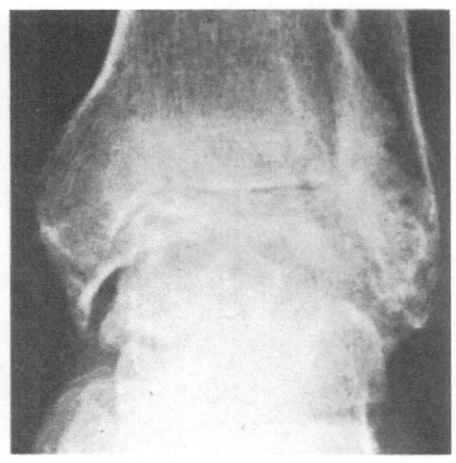

31/b

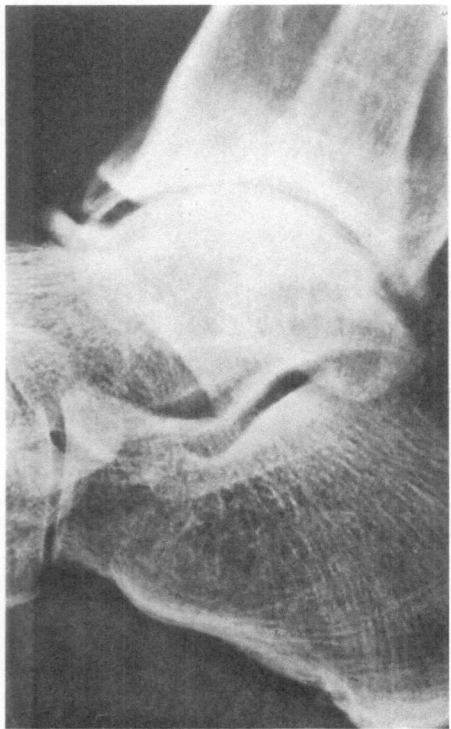

31/c

Fig. 31. P. J., haemophilia A

(a–c) Severe arthrosis deformans in both ankles. The articular surfaces have almost completely regenerated. Coarse subchondral sclerosis in the joints

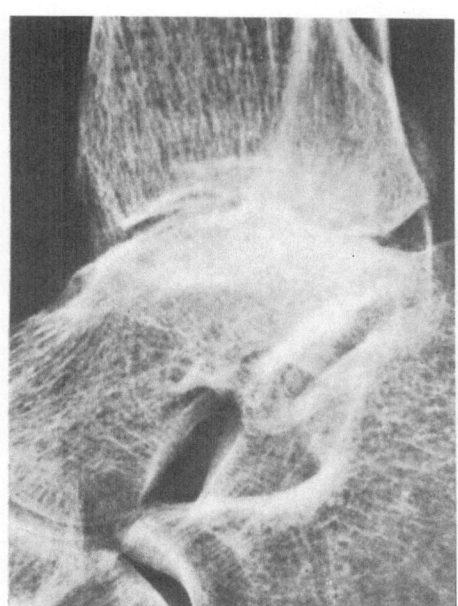

Fig. 32. S. J., 25 years, haemophilia A

(a, b) Chronic atrophy. Flattened trochlea of the talus

32/a

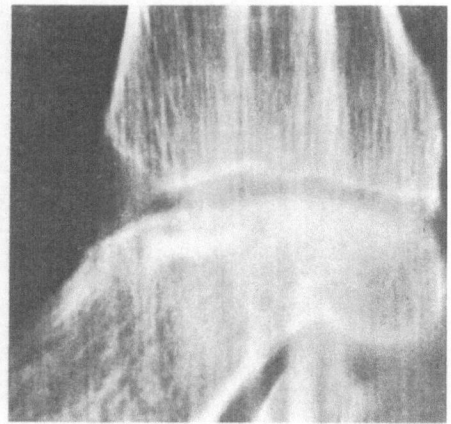

32/b

Fig. 33. L. J., 26 years, haemophilia A

Besides the alterations of the talocrural articulation, the coarse arthropathy of the posterior talocalcaneal articulation is striking

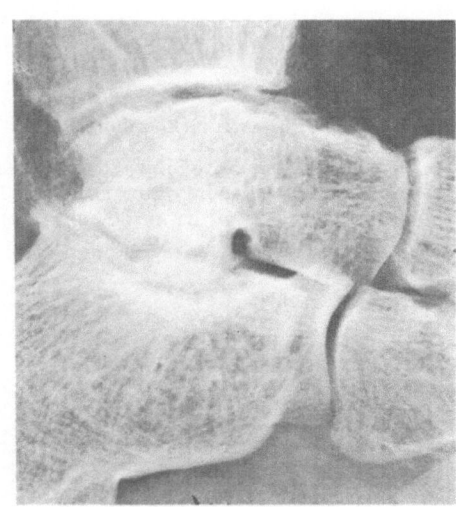

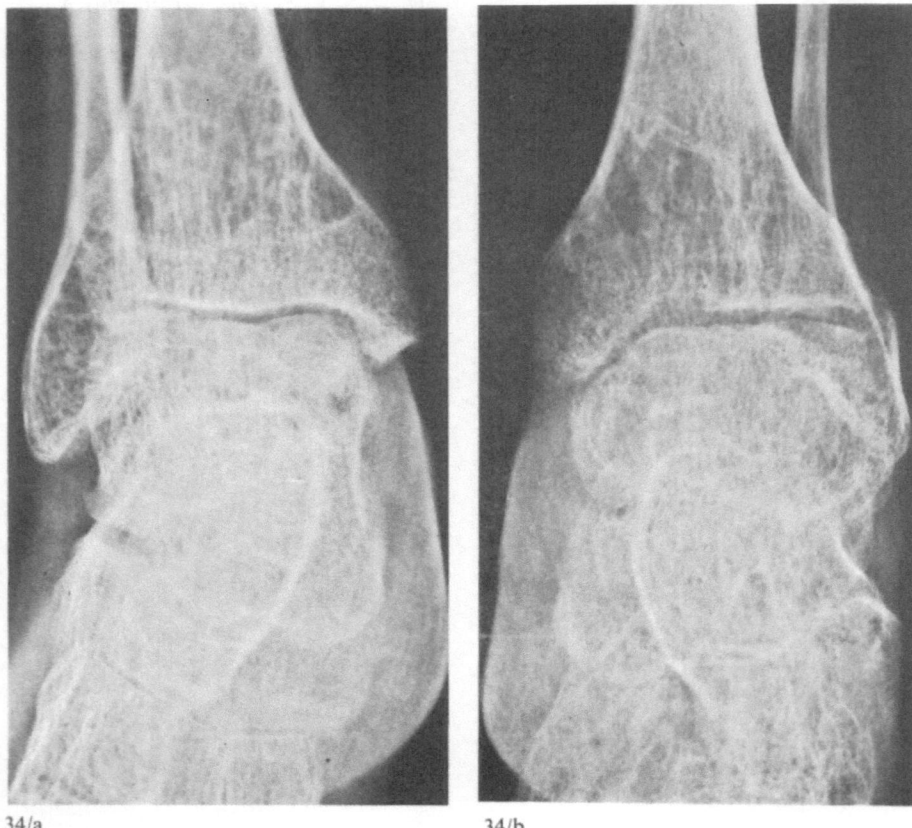

34/a   34/b

Fig. 34. H. S., 30 years, haemophilia B

(a, b) Classical picture of the regressive stage. Uniform, extensive atrophy, characteristic rearrangement in the spongy bone structure. The surface of the left talus has become spherical. Note the hypoplasia of the metadiaphysis of the left tibia

Hip

Haemarthrosis

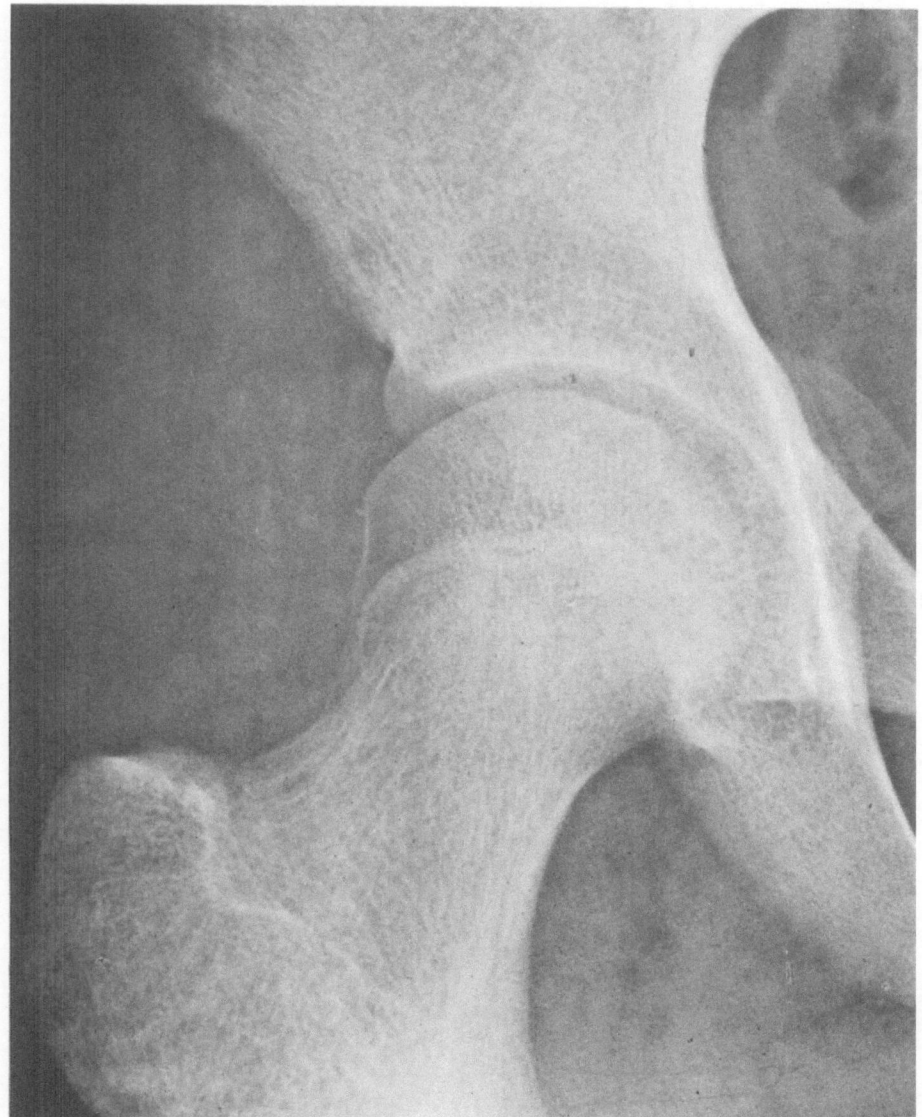

Fig. 35. H. Z., 14 years, haemophilia A

Slight coxa valga position. The lateral edge of the femoral epiphysis is flattened; intact contour. The changes are considered to be due to posthaemarthrotic dystrophy or resorption

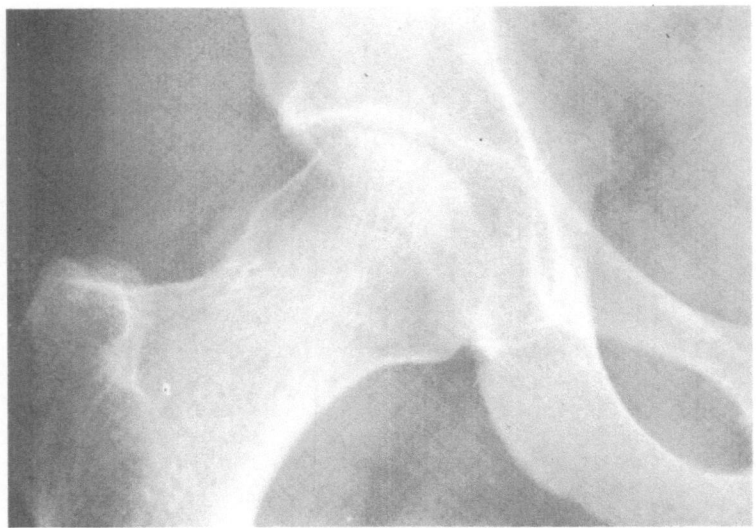

Fig. 36. H. S., 30 years, haemophilia B

Considerable flattening of the lateral edge of the femur. A lentil-sized compact island in the neck of the femur and in the acetabulum. The collodiaphyseal angle is normal. Note the slight hypoplasia of the femoral head

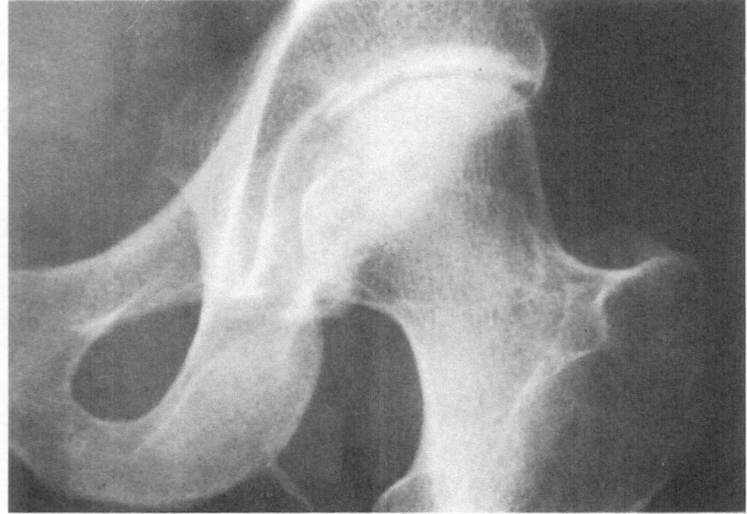

Fig. 37. Sz. J., 35 years, haemophilia A

Coxa valga, dysplastic head of the femur with flat and steep lateral edge

Fig. 38. B. J., 18 years, haemophilia A

Marked coxa valga position. Laterally from the fovea capitis the contour is flattened over a short distance. Fine subchondral resorption medially

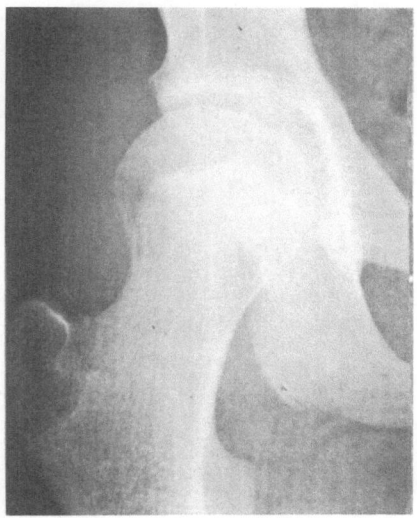

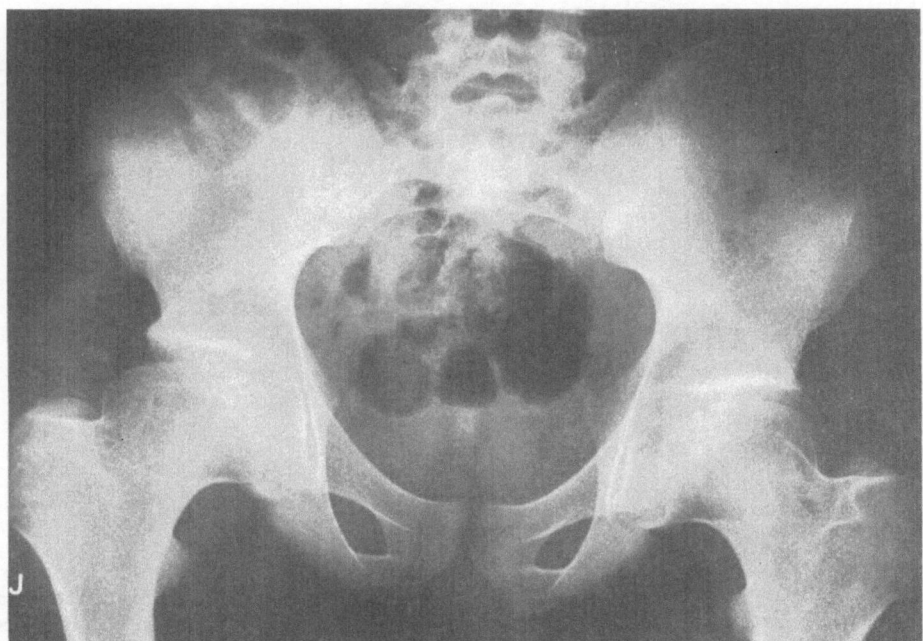

Fig. 39. Sz. V., 19 years, haemophilia A

Coarse, mushroom-like flattening of the head of the femur on the right side. Intact articular surfaces, normal joint space. The course of Perthes' disease has been regular, the articular cartilages have remained intact

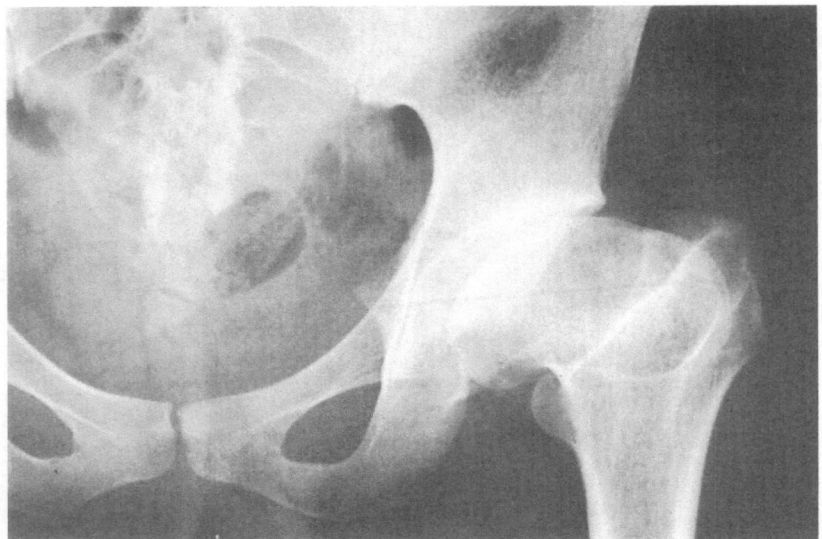

40/a

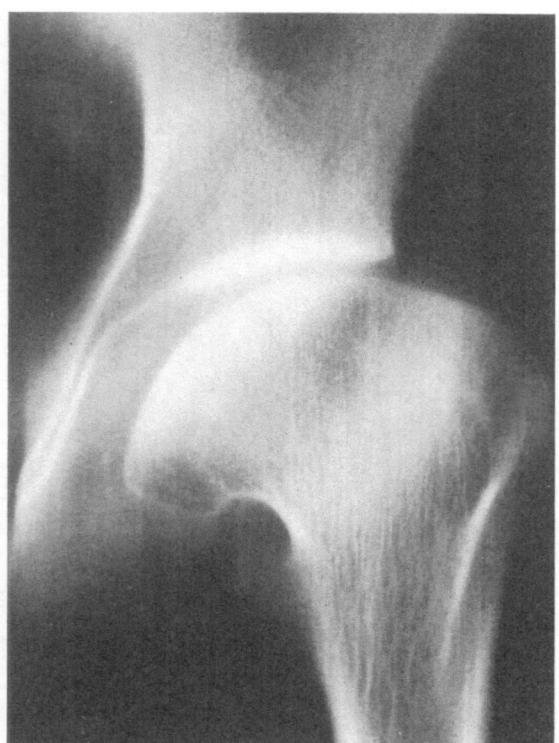

40/b

Fig. 40. D. V., 21 years, haemophilia A

(a) Coxa vara, marked mushroomlike deformation of the head of the femur, indicating an earlier Perthes' disease

(b) The tomogram displays the intact contour of the articular surface

98

Panarthritis

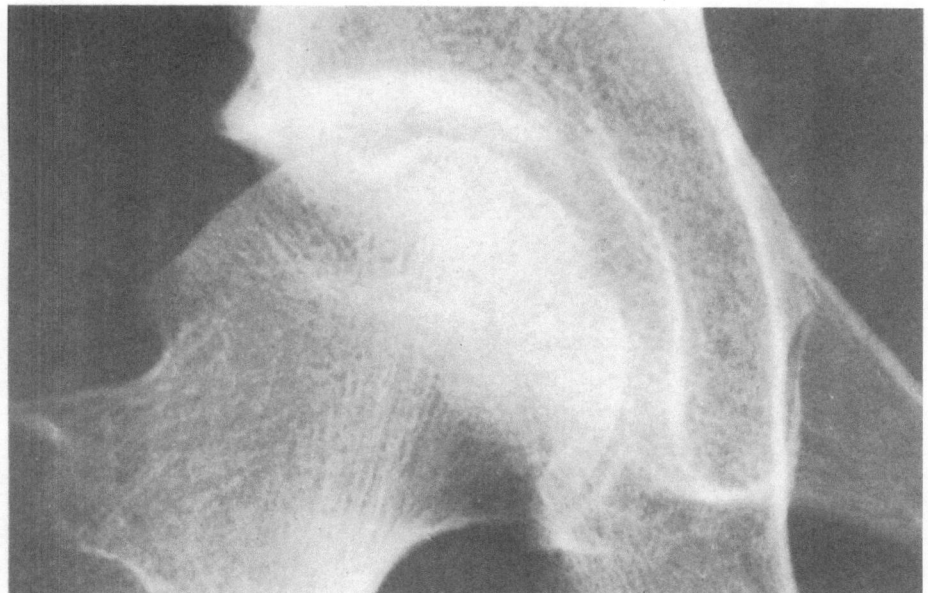

Fig. 41. F. G., 26 years, haemophilia A

The highest point of the otherwise regular head of the femur is pitted, its border is sclerotic

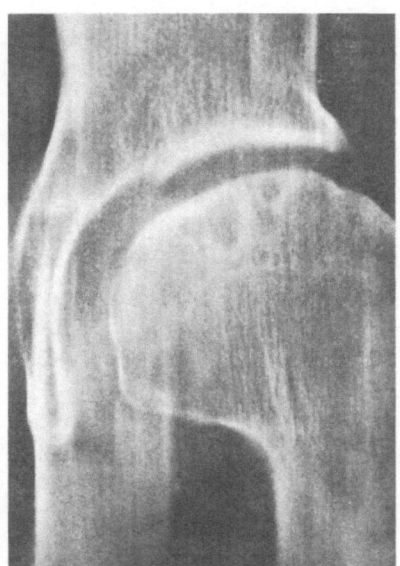

Fig. 42. N. Gy., 39 years, haemophilia A

Lentil- to pea-sized cysts under the irregular articular surface

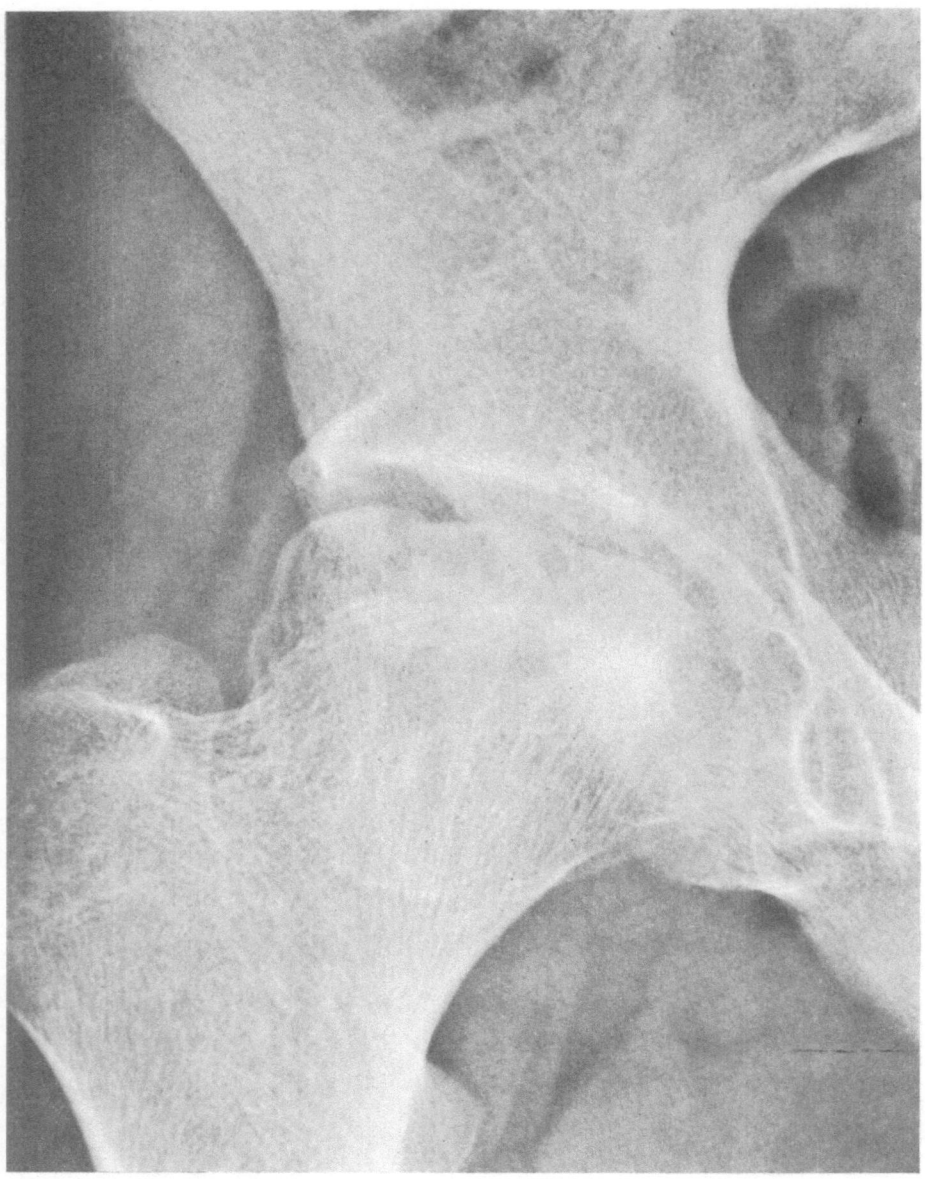

43/a

Fig. 43. Sz. B., 16 years, haemophilia A

Mushroom-shaped, flattened head of the femur, the shape of the acetabulum has changed accordingly

(a) Uneven femoral articular surface

100

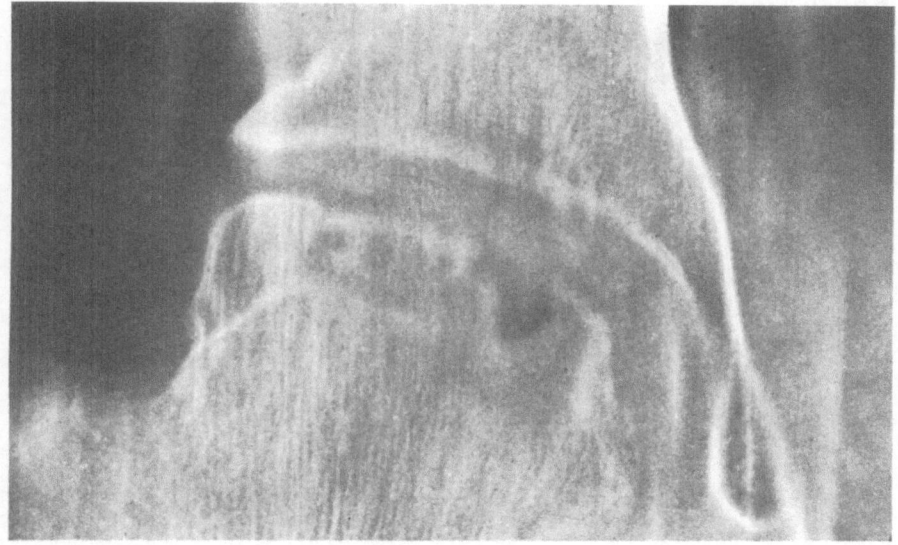

43/b

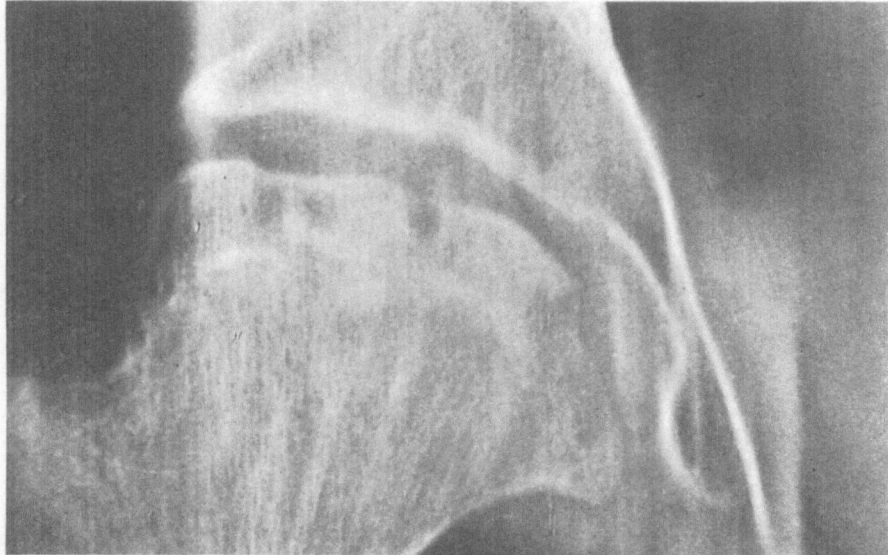

43/c

Fig. 43

(b, c) Tomograms: subchondral cysts, above some of them the articular surface is pitted, others communicate widely with the joint space

101

Regression

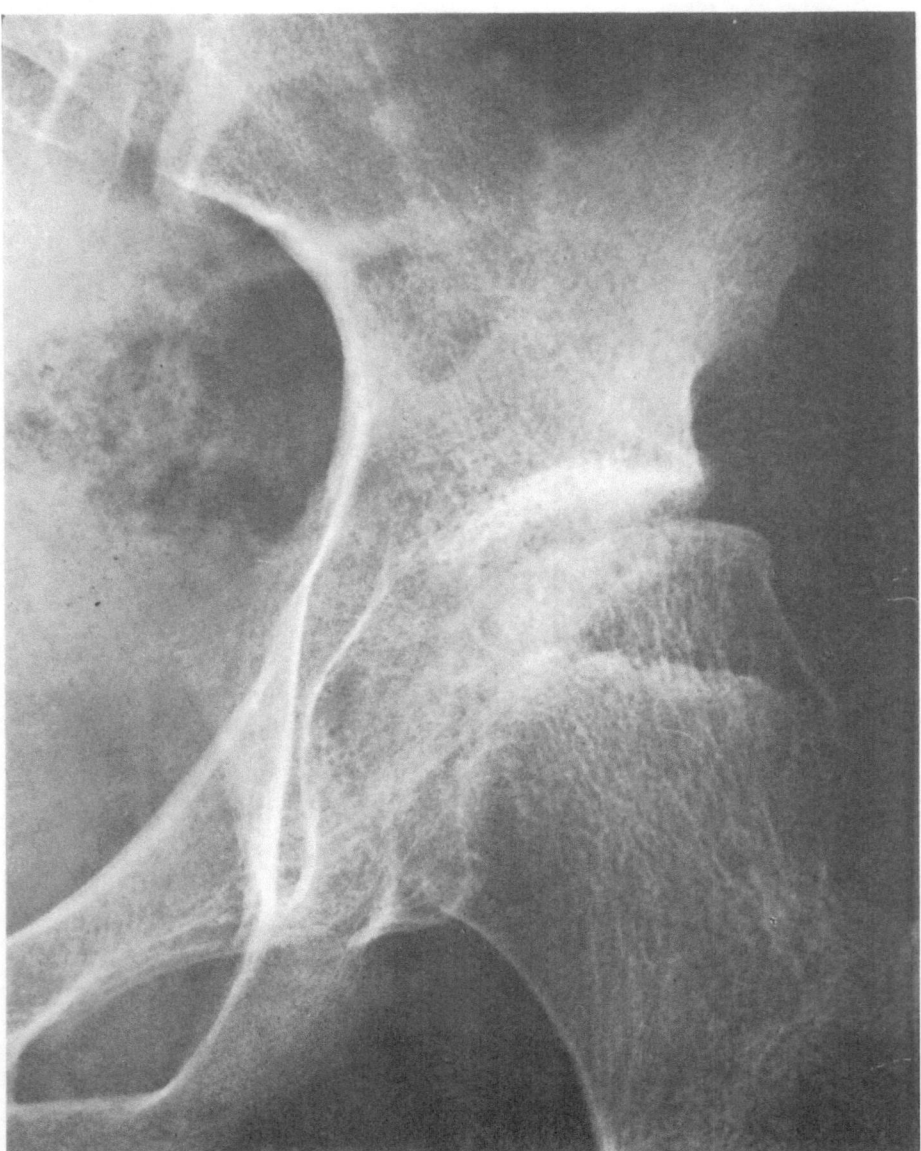

44/a

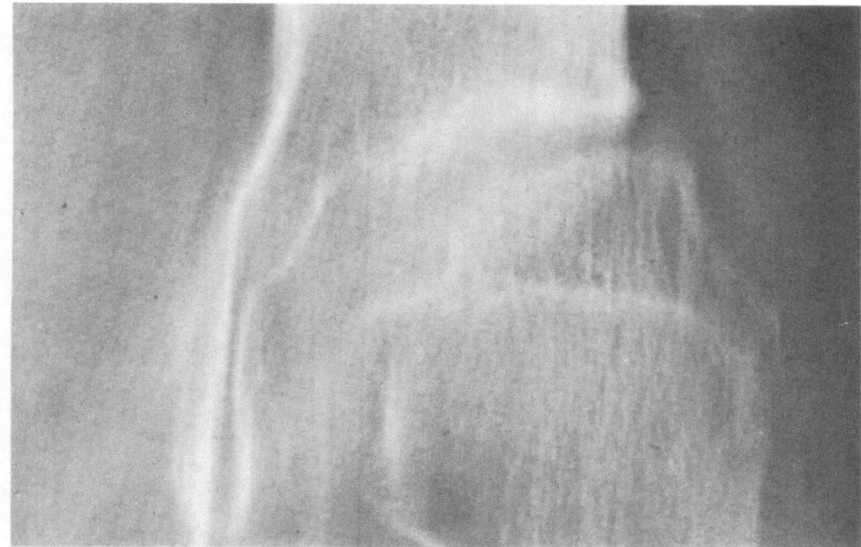

44/b

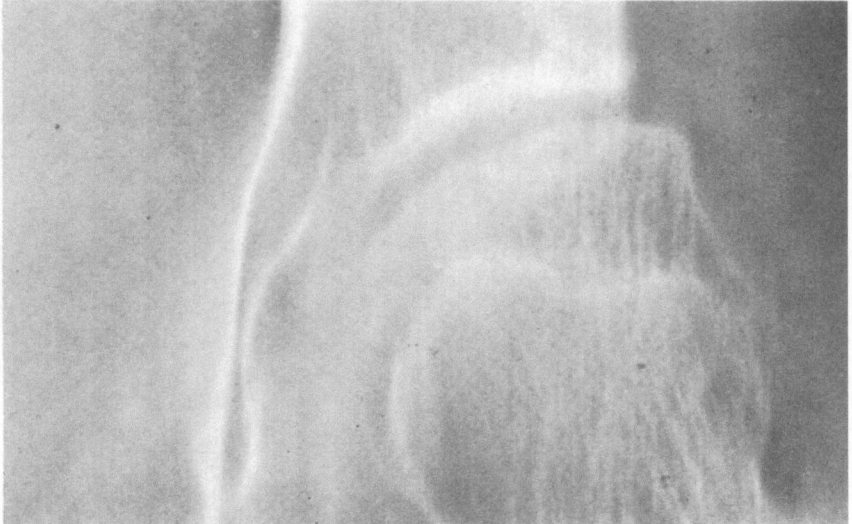

44/c

Fig. 44. R. B., 14 years, haemophilia A

(a–c) Left side: chronic atrophy, lateral contour of the femoral head is flattened. Irregular articular surfaces. Characteristic signs of panarthritis still prevail

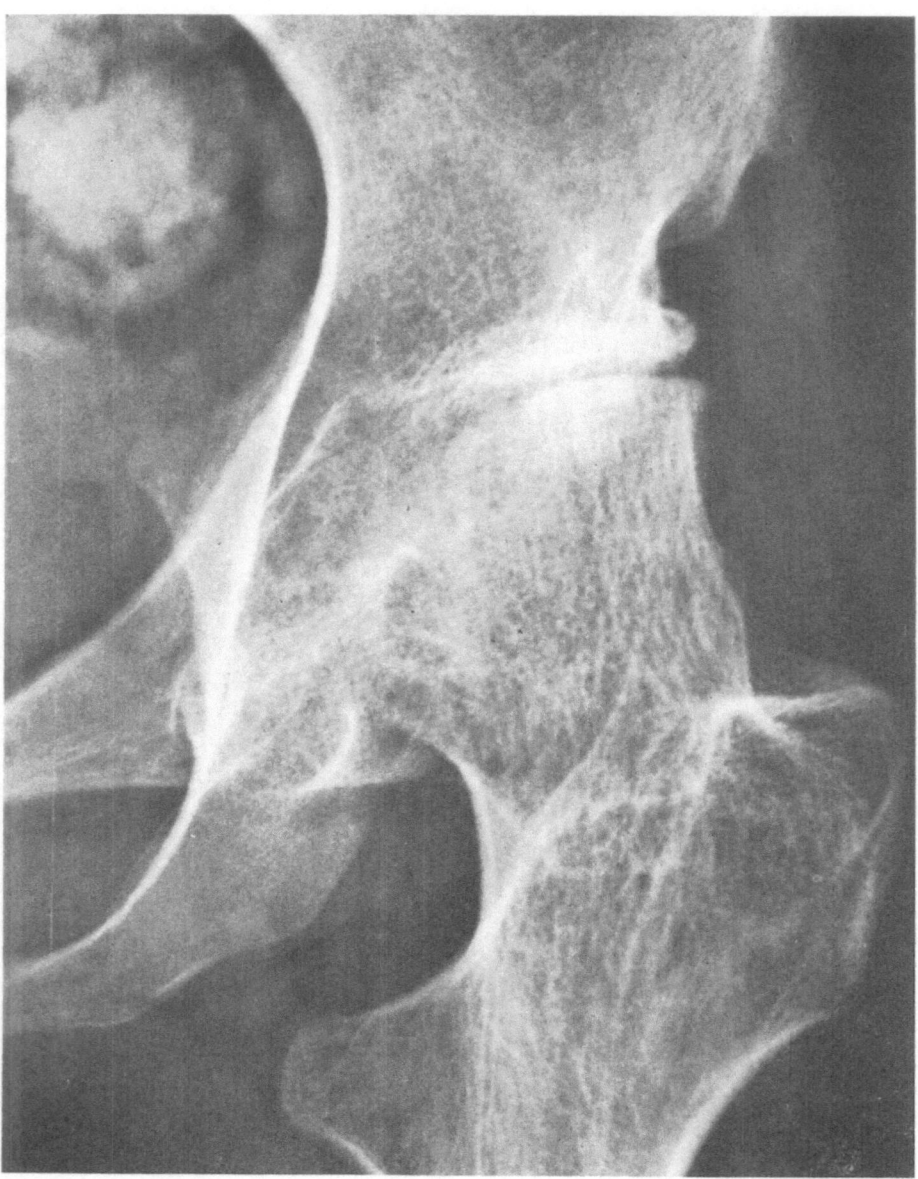

44/d

Fig. 44

(d) The same hip 5 years later. The joint space of the left hip is narrowed; as a result, arthrotic lipping has formed at the lateral edges of the articular surfaces. The structure indicates marked chronic atrophy. Subchondrally a few large cysts are still visible

104

Elbow

Haemarthrosis

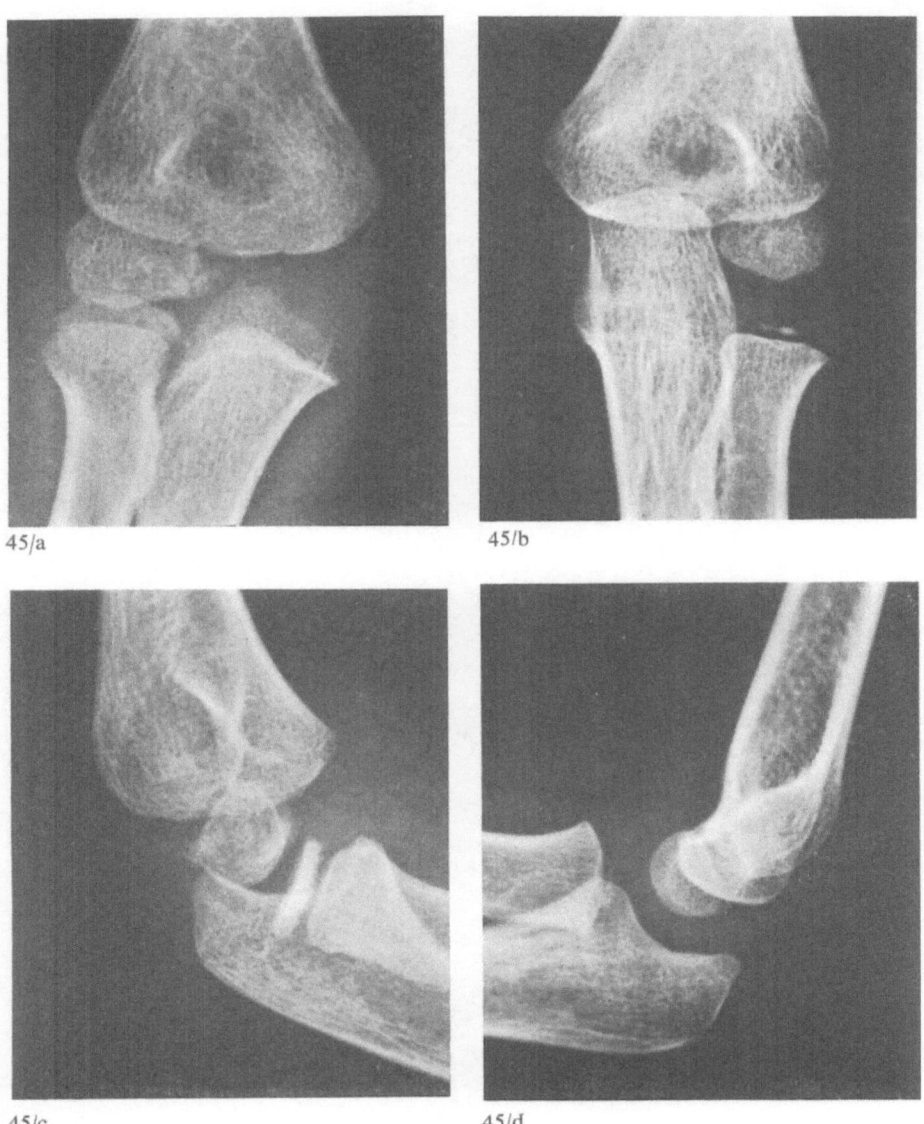

45/a

45/b

45/c

45/d

Fig. 45. E. J., 6 years, haemophilia A

(a, b) Recurrent haemarthroses in the right elbow. Note the difference between the epiphyses: on the right side the epiphysis of the capitulum of the humerus and of the head of the radius are relatively more developed than on the left side

(c, d) Lateral view: particularly the more developed head the of radius can be well noted

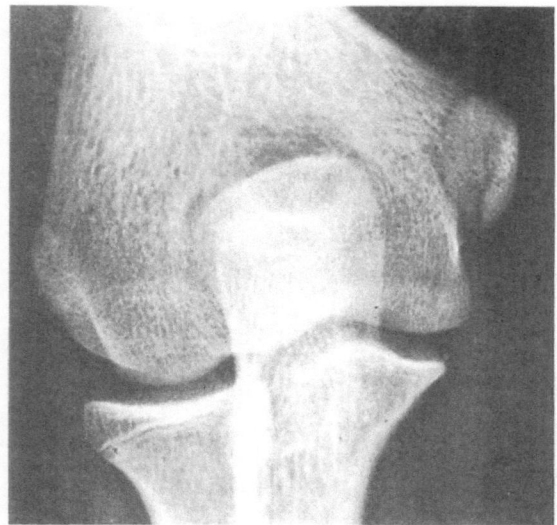

46/a

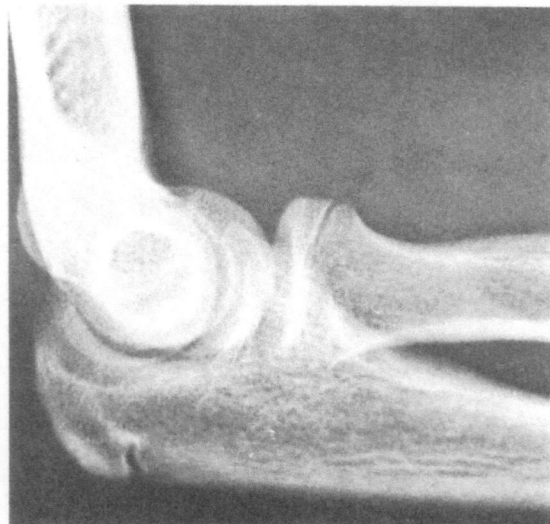

46/b

Fig. 46. Sz. B., 16 years, haemophilia A

(a–d) Right elbow: normal. Left elbow: prematurely ossified apophysis of the ulnar epicondyle of the humerus; there is a large supratrochlear foramen. On the affected side the epiphysis of the head of the radius has fused, on the right side it has not

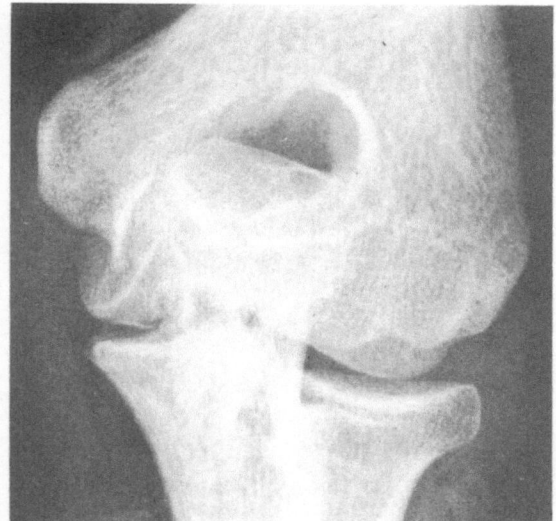

46/c

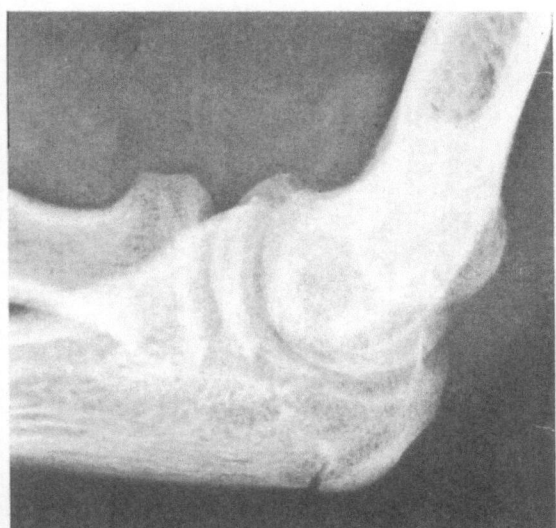

46/d

107

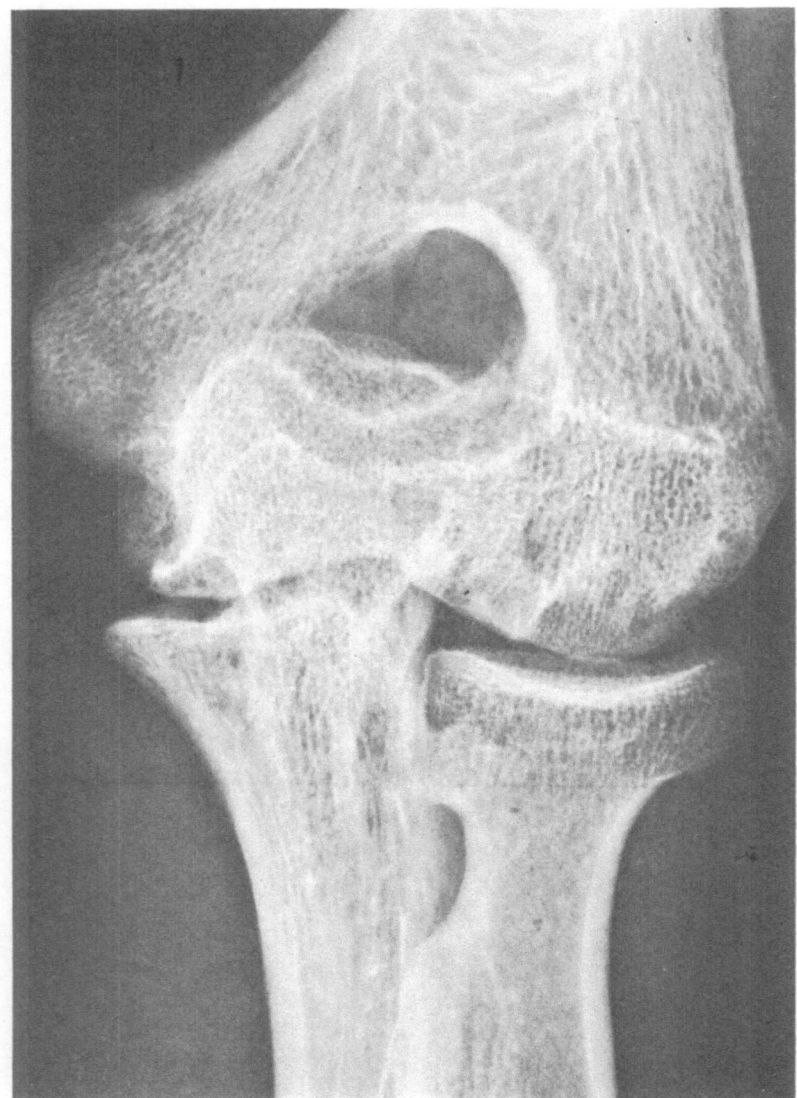

46/e

Fig. 46

(e, f) Direct magnification: the fine signs of focal subchondral lysis are just visible. Fine unevenness of the articular surface

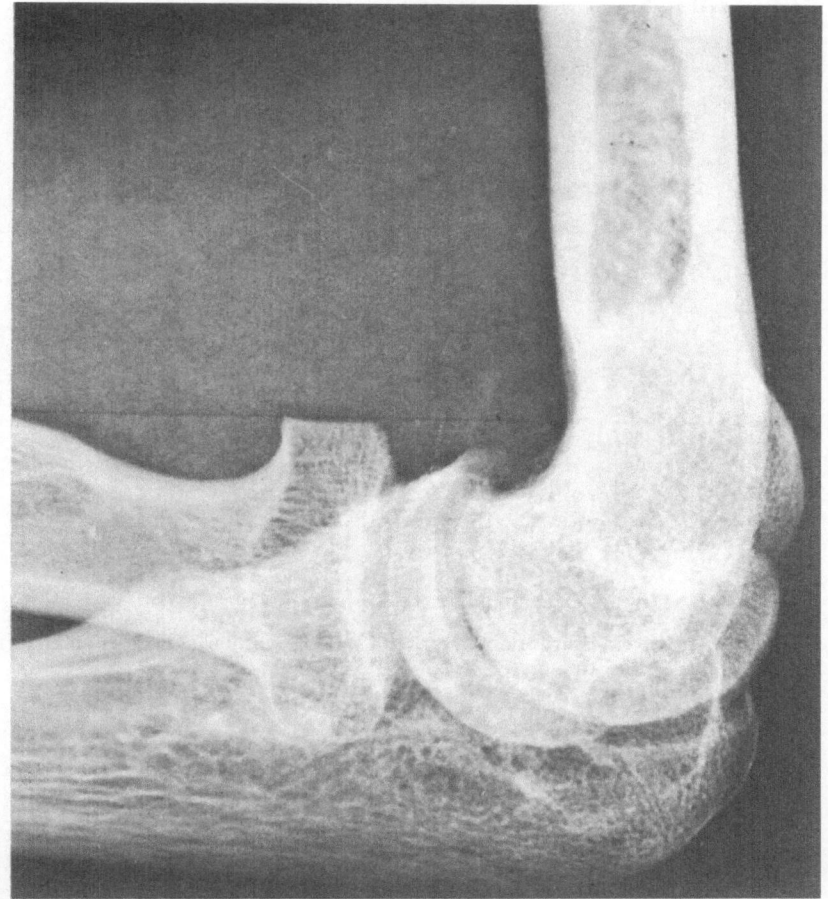

46/f

Panarthritis

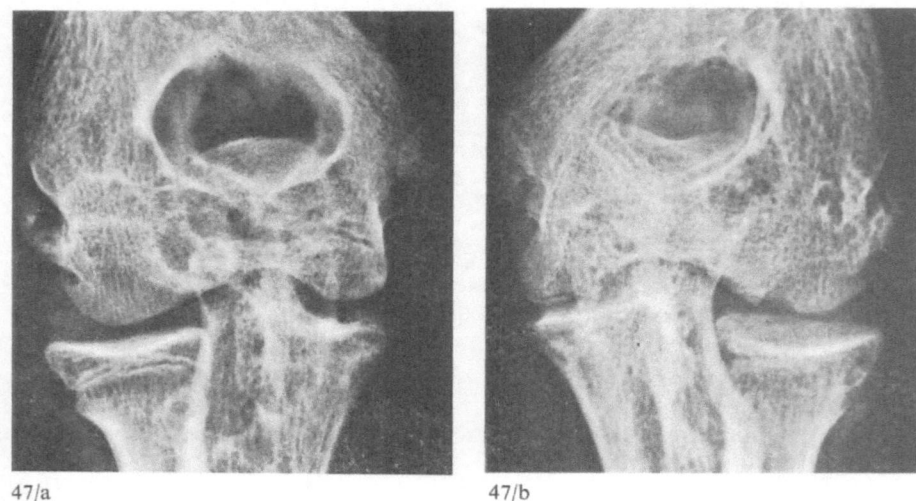

47/a   47/b

Fig. 47. B. B., 12 years, haemophilia A

(a, b) Large supratrochlear foramina on both sides. Slightly irregular articular surfaces. Rarified bone substance with lytic foci

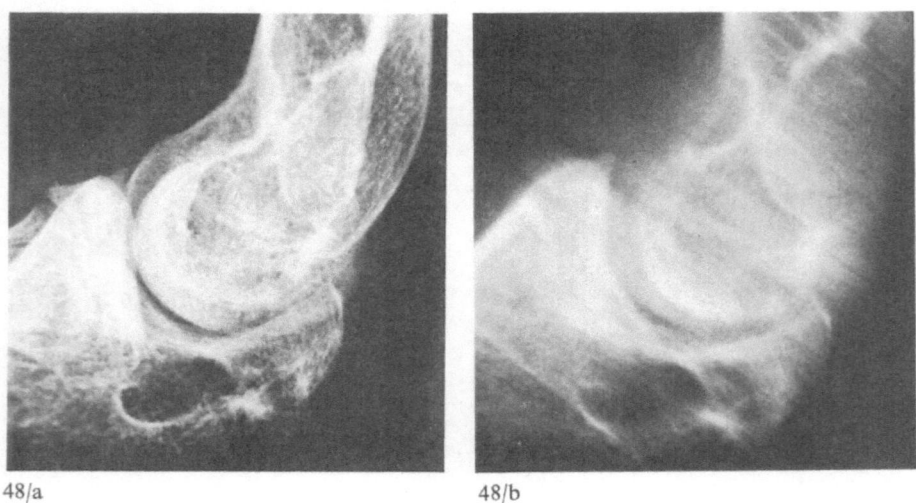

48/a   48/b

Fig. 48. F. I., 14 years, haemophilia A

(a, b) Lateral view: a single bean-sized cyst in the olecranon. The tomogram reveals a marked unevenness of the articular surfaces. The olecranon fossa and the coronoid fossa are deeply excavated

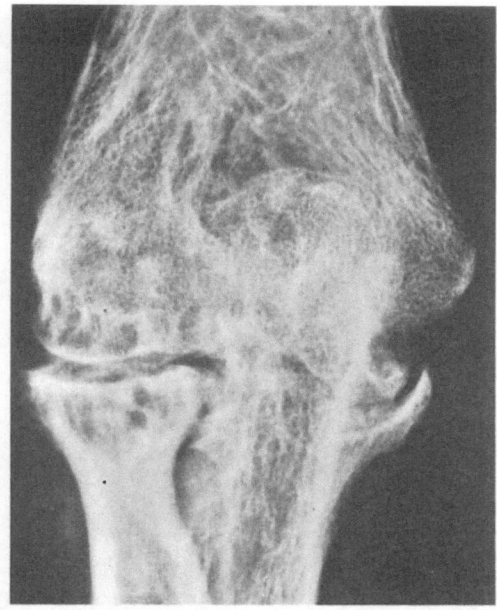

49/a

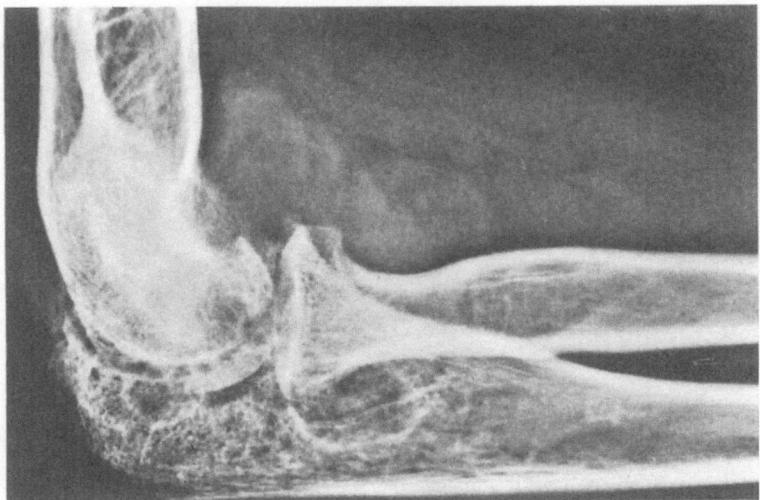

49/b

Fig. 49. S. J., 23 years, haemophilia A

(a, b) The articular space is narrowed. Under the articular surfaces a string of cysts is visible. The lateral edge of the olecranon's articular surface is prominent, opposite it, as a result of resorption, the ulnar epicondyle of the humerus, the articular surface of the humeral trochlea, is deeply undermined

111

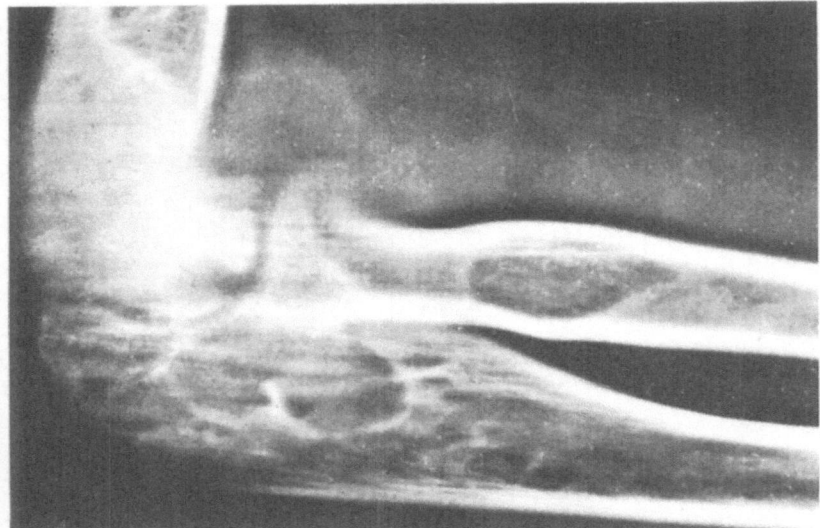

49/c

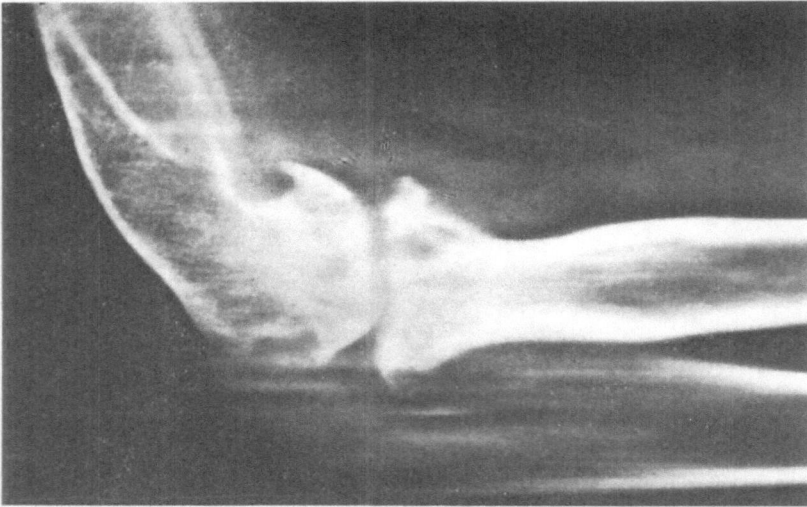

49/d

Fig. 49

(c) Lateral tomogram in the depth of the ulna. A segmented cyst of date-stone size is visible in the olecranon. In this layer the radial capitulum humeri forms a beak-like process

(d) In a more radial layer the humeroradial articulation is well visible. The contour of the capitulum is flattened, the volar and dorsal edges are both deeply undermined, forming pseudoosteophytes. Pea-sized cyst in the head of the radius, communicating with the joint space

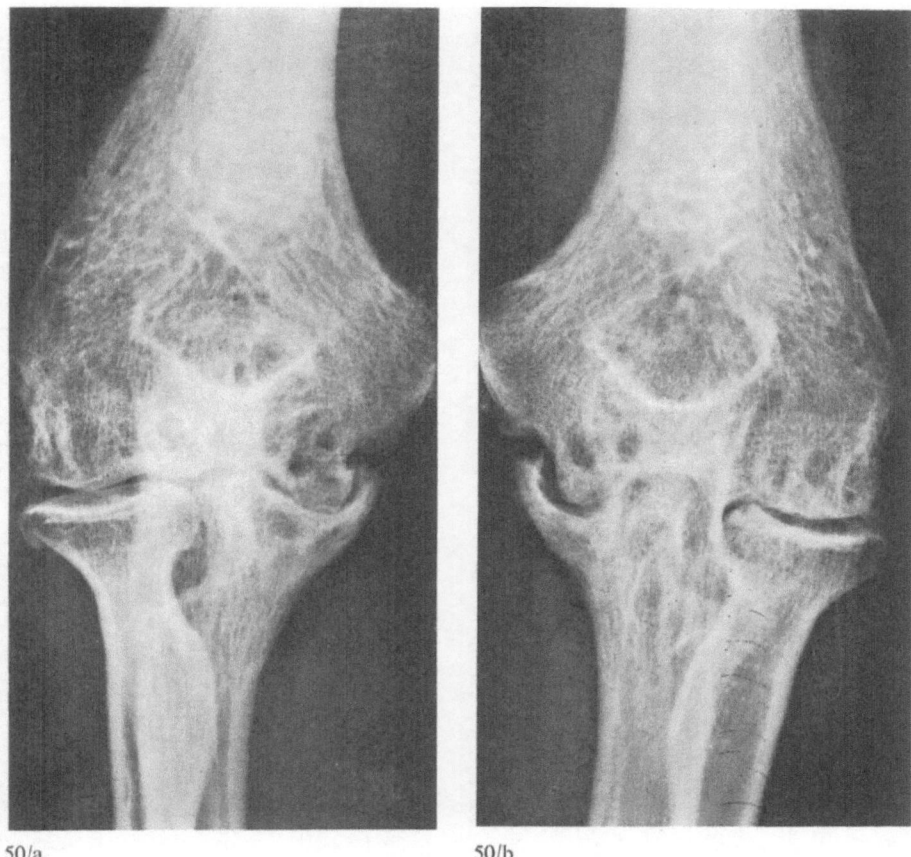

50/a   50/b

Fig. 50. S. J., 30 years, haemophilia B

(a, b) Narrowed joint spaces, numerous subchondral cysts. The lateral half of the articular surface of the olecranon is destroyed, its horn-shaped edge supports the ulnar epicondyle of the humerus

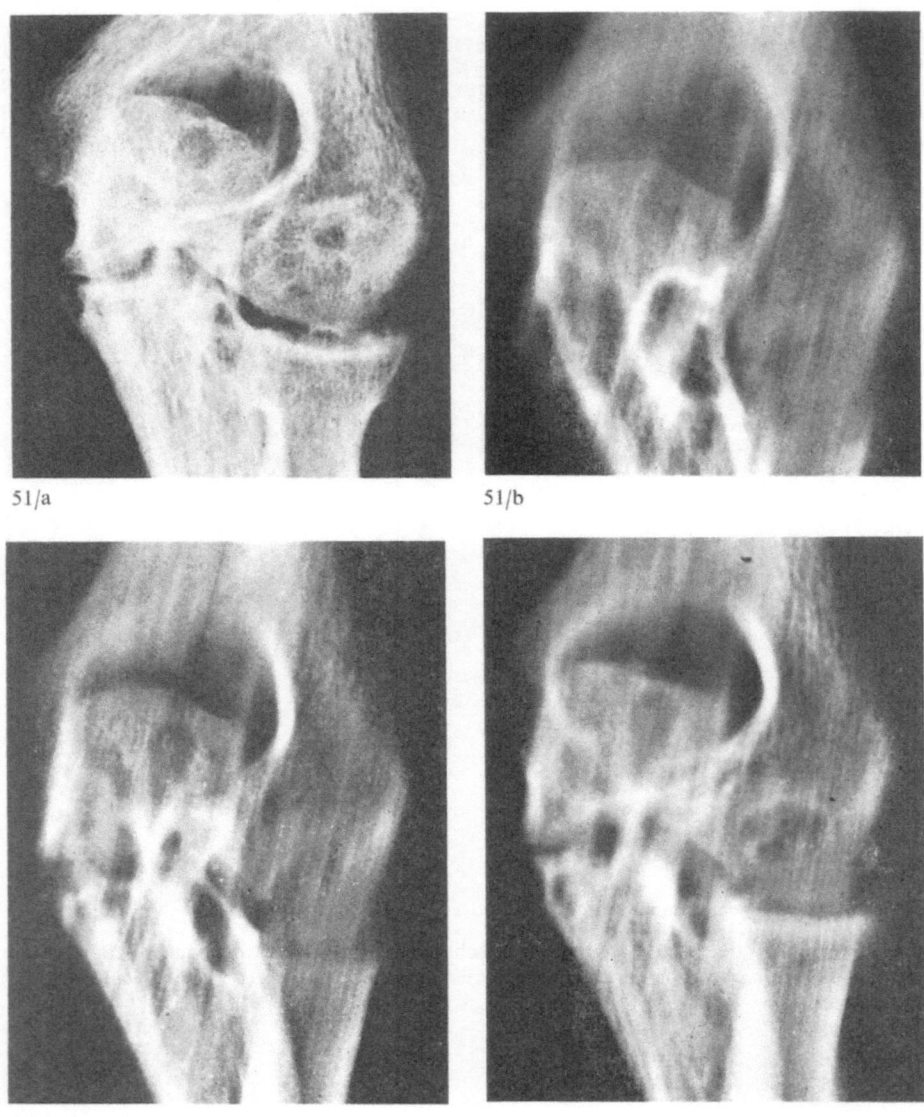

51/a

51/b

51/c

51/d

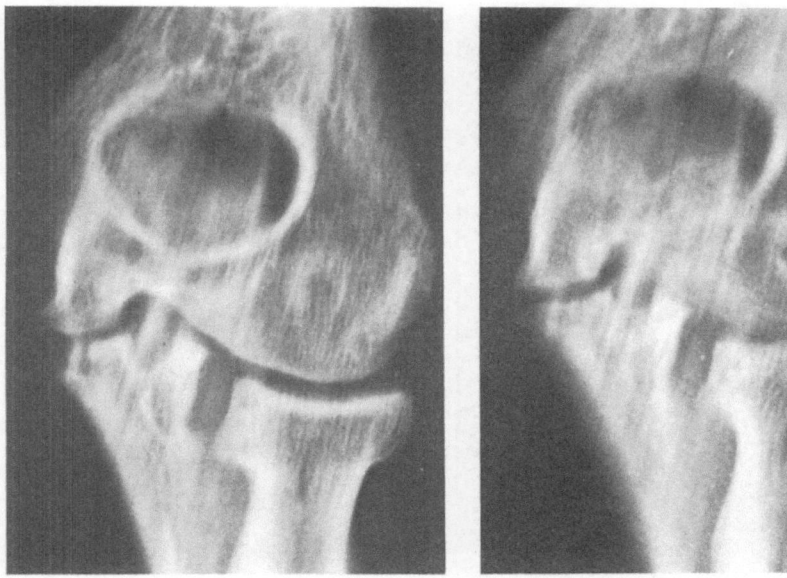

51/e 51/f

Fig. 51. H. Gy., 15 years, haemophilia A

(a–f) Destroyed articular surfaces, large supratrochlear foramen. Tomograms made at 1.5, 2, 2.5, 3, 3.5 cm depths demonstrate in detail the destruction of the articular surface and the cysts variable in location and size

8*

115

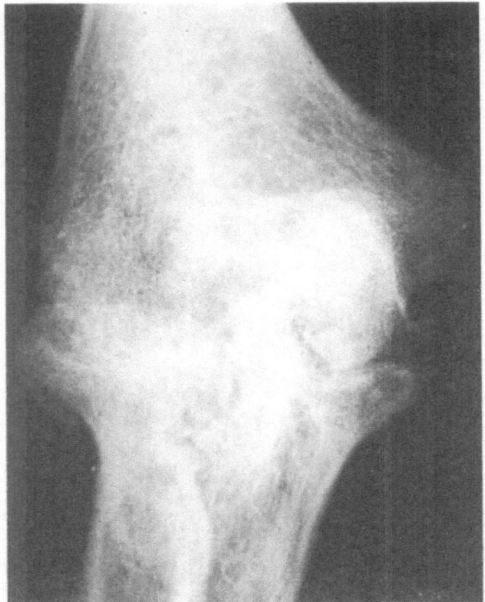

52/a

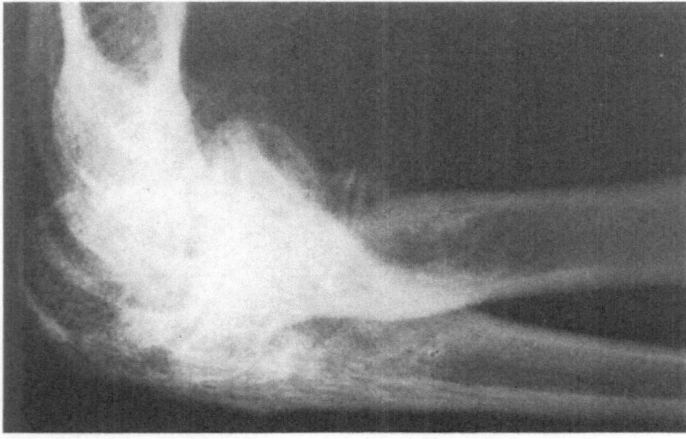

52/b

Fig. 52. P. F., 20 years, haemophilia A

(a, b) Extremely serious destruction, massive sclerosis. The over-developed head of the radius is flattened. Note the Looser's zone on the volar part of the neck of the radius. The conductor crest of the olecranon is prominent as a result of the destruction of the articular surfaces of the olecranon. The picture is similar to that seen in syringomyelia

116

Regression

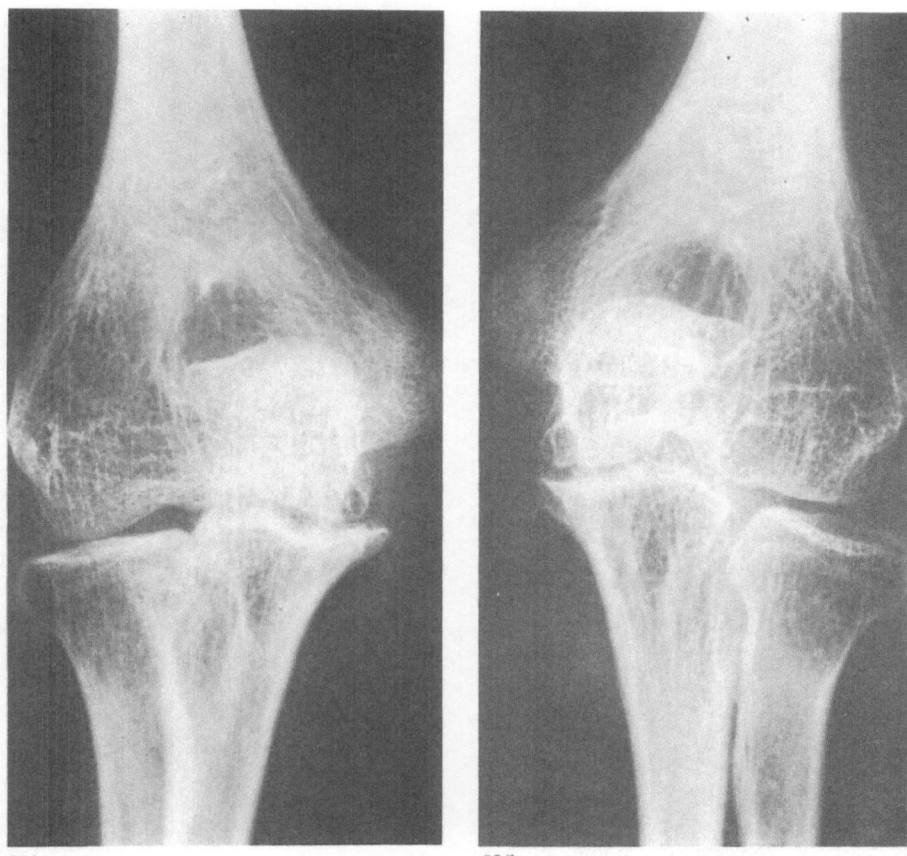

53/a   53/b

Fig. 53. R. B., 14 years, haemophilia A

(a, b) The classical stage of regression has developed at a relatively early age. All epiphyseal ossification centres have fused early indicating previous acute processes. The bones are slightly deformed, their structure displays the typical features of chronic atrophy. Cysts occur sporadically. Irregular articular surfaces, distinct contours. The left radius is curved

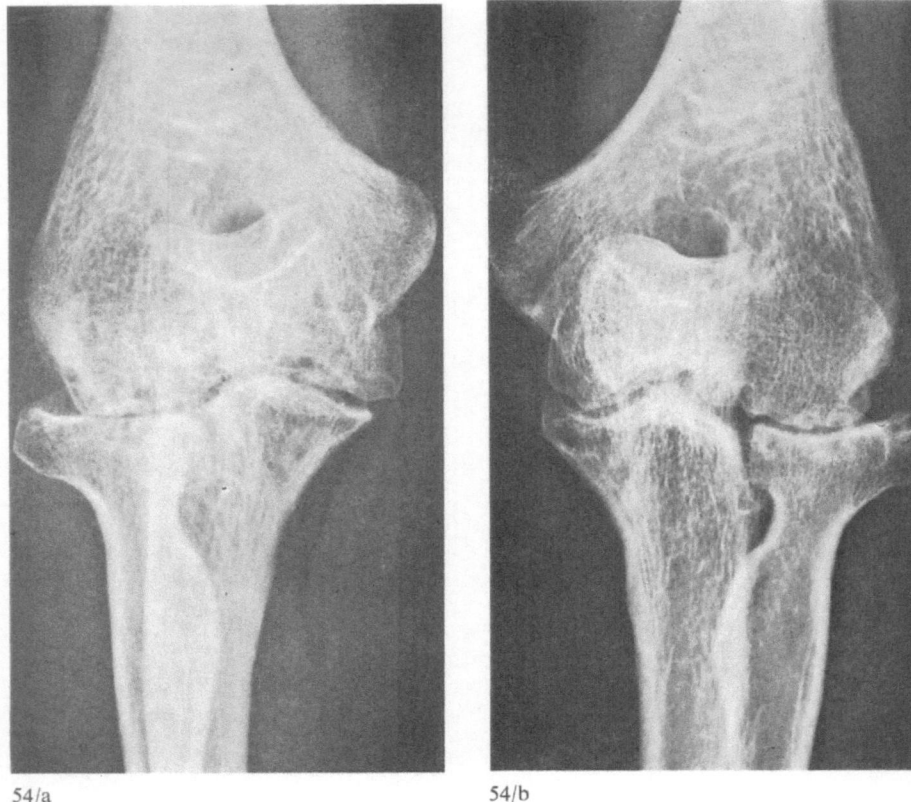

54/a   54/b

Fig. 54. F. T., 26 years, haemophilia A

(a, b) Markedly narrowed joint space, irregular but distinct contours. The bowl-shaped widening of the head of the radius far overlapping the lateral edge of the radial capitulum humeri is typical

Fig. 56. B. L., 30 years, haemophilia A

(a, b) Supratrochlear foramen in the affected right joint. Deformed articular surfaces. Marked arthrosis in the radioulnar articulation. Intact conditions on the left side

118

Fig. 55. D. V. 17 years, haemophilia A

Deformed articular surfaces, slight atrophy. The epiphyseal centres have partially fused. Numerous small cysts in the olecranon

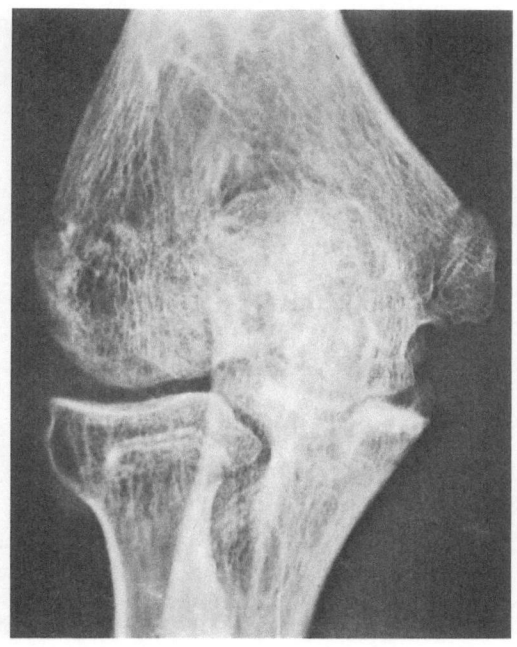

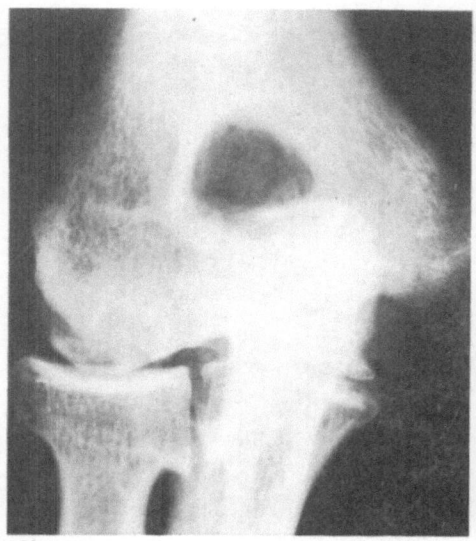

56/a

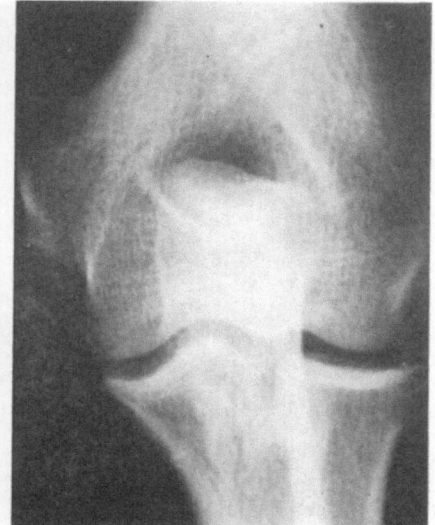

56/b

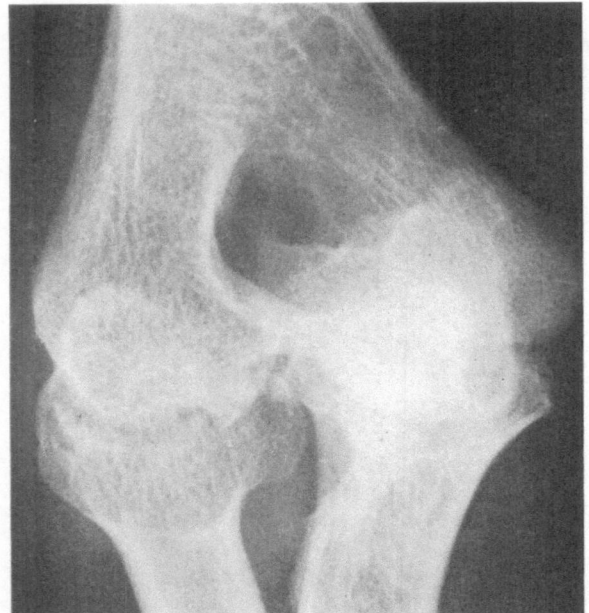

57/a

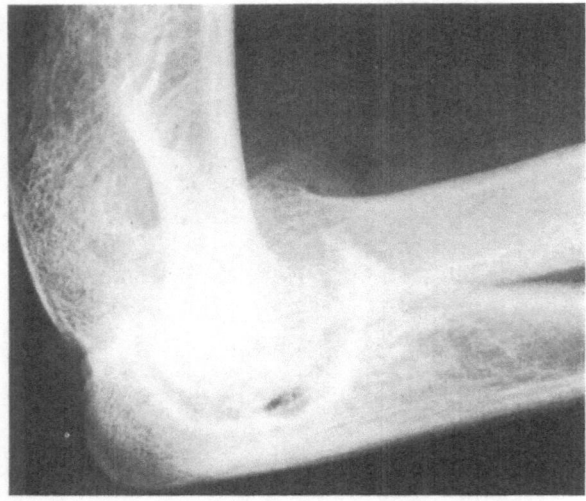

57/b

Fig. 57. B. I., 18 years, haemophilia A

(a, b) A–P and lateral view

120

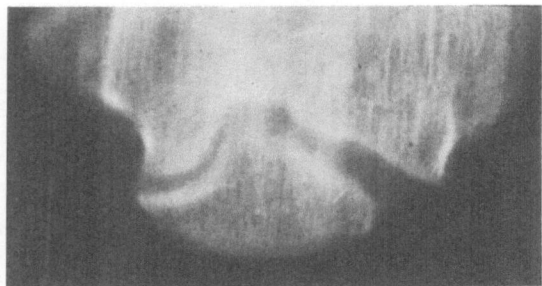

57/c

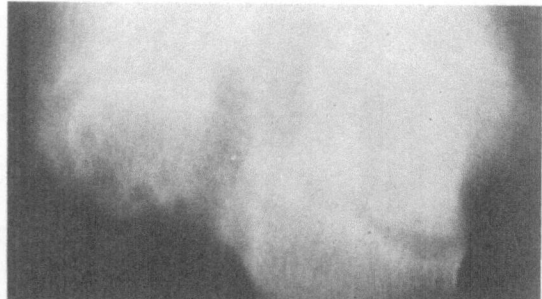

57/d

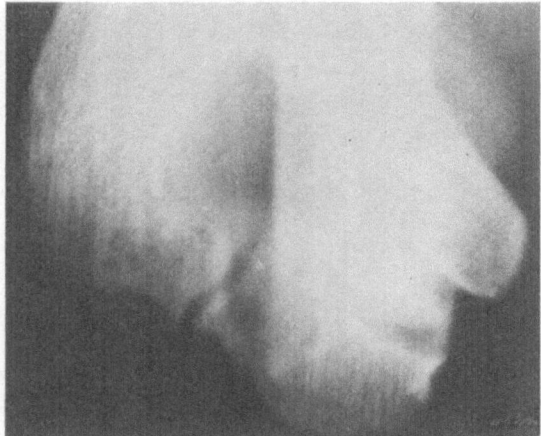

57/e

(c–e) The three tomograms have been made in axial position. Note, besides the usual alterations, the penetration of the humeral trochlea into the deeply excavated olecranon. The conductor crest of the olecranon cuts through the trochlea and penetrates the trochlear foramen of the humerus

121

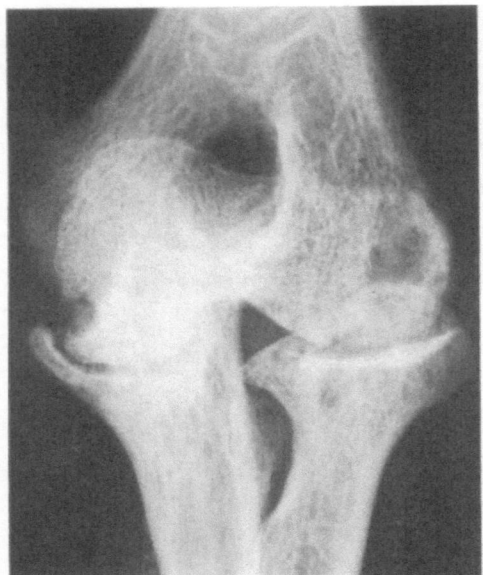

58/a

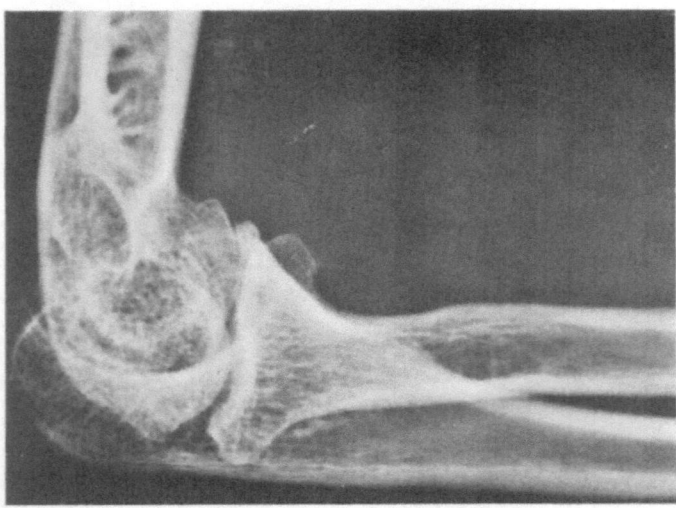

58/b

Fig. 58. H. S., 30 years, haemophilia B

(a, b) The head of the radius is severely deformed, flattened. The trochlea deeply penetrates into the ulnar articular surface of the olecranon. Note the deep erosion on the external contour of the latter, and the excrescence on the edge of the ulna opposite it

Shoulder

Haemarthrosis

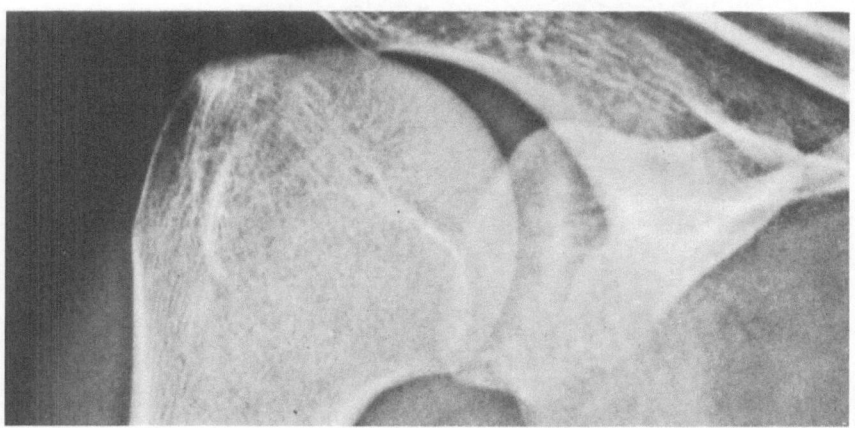

Fig. 59. Sz. R., 21 years, haemophilia A

Severe arthropathy in numerous joints. In the right shoulder a number of haem-arthrotic episodes have occurred. Humerus varus, striking parrot-beak-shaped epi-physis

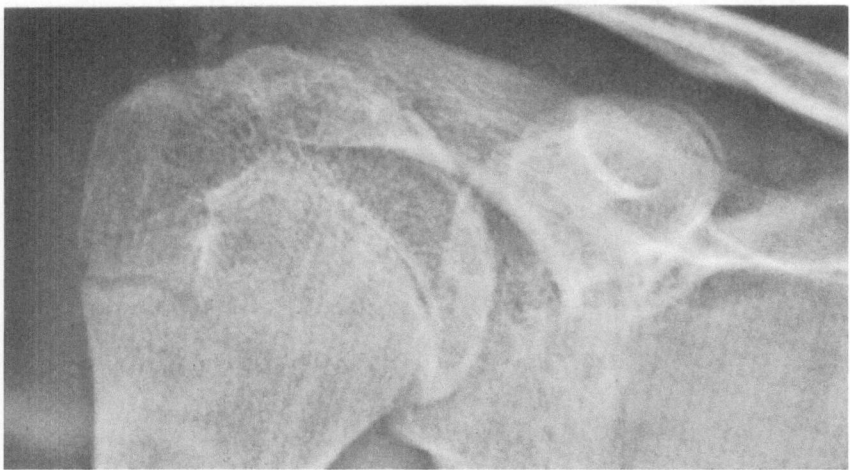

Fig. 60. P. J., 17 years, haemophilia A

Repeated episodes of haemarthrosis in the right shoulder. Marked humerus varus. The epiphyseal structure is rarified and atrophic, the joint contour is uneven, its shape is parrot-beak-like

Panarthritis

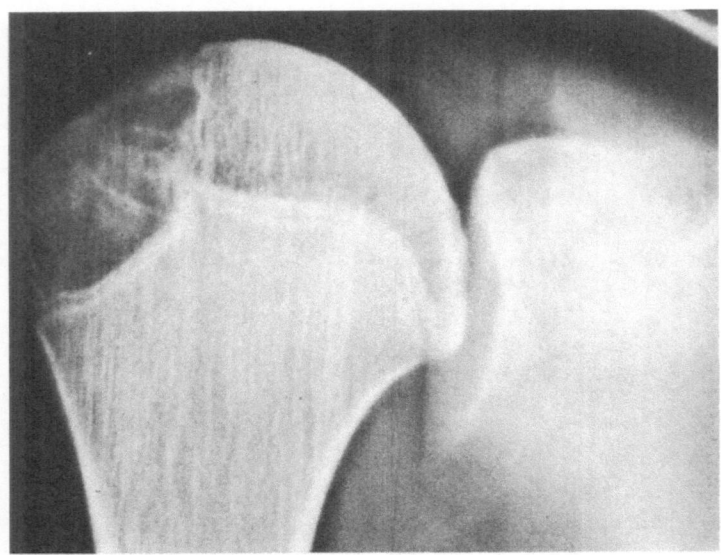

Fig. 61. N. B., 14 years, haemophilia A

The articular contour of the parrot-beak-shaped process of the humeral epiphysis is irregular. Marked cystic atrophy on the greater tuberosity

Fig. 62. G. J., 23 years,
haemophilia A

(a–c) Numerous lentil-sized cysts
under the glenoid fossa. At the
edges of the articular surface of
the head of the humerus bean-
to peanut-sized cysts. The tomograms display an indented articular surface contour over the
cysts

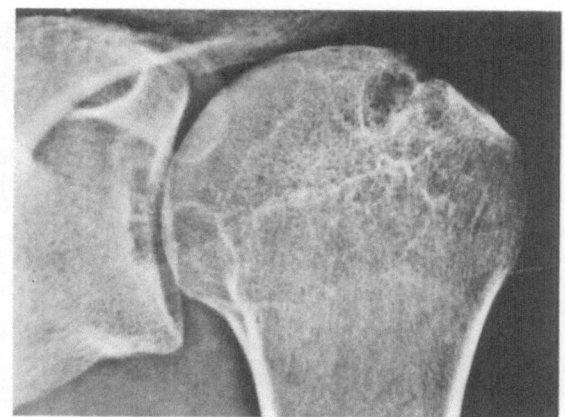

62/a

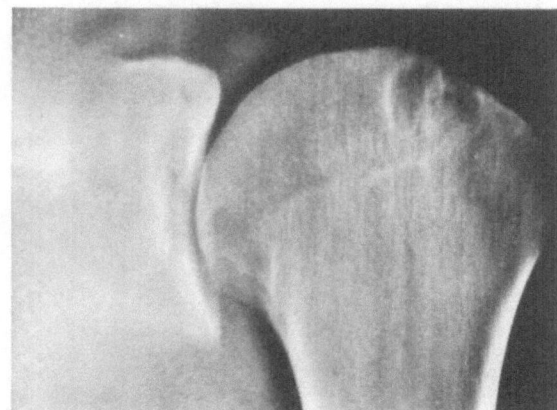

62/b

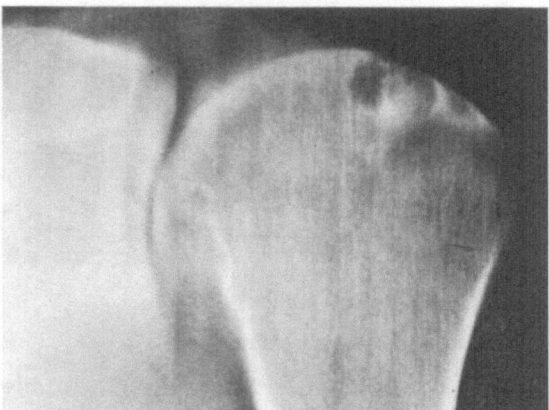

62/c

125

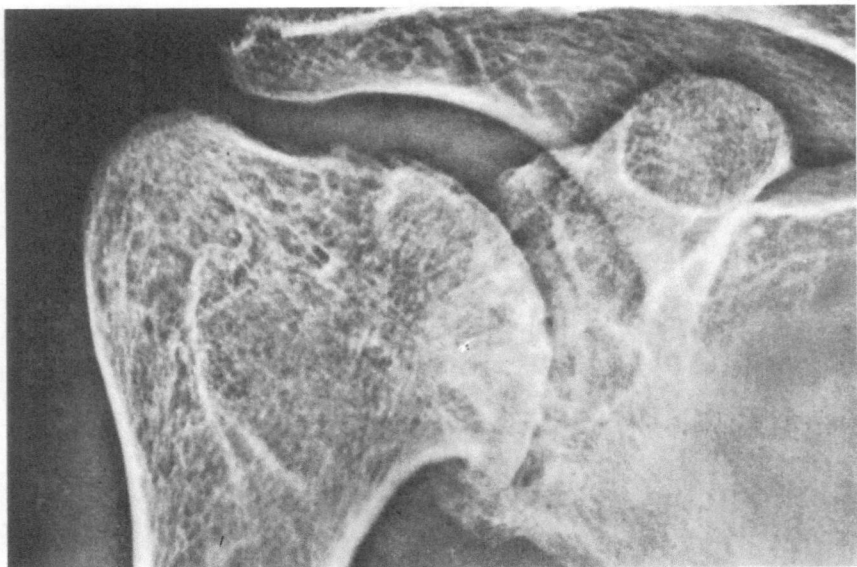

63/a

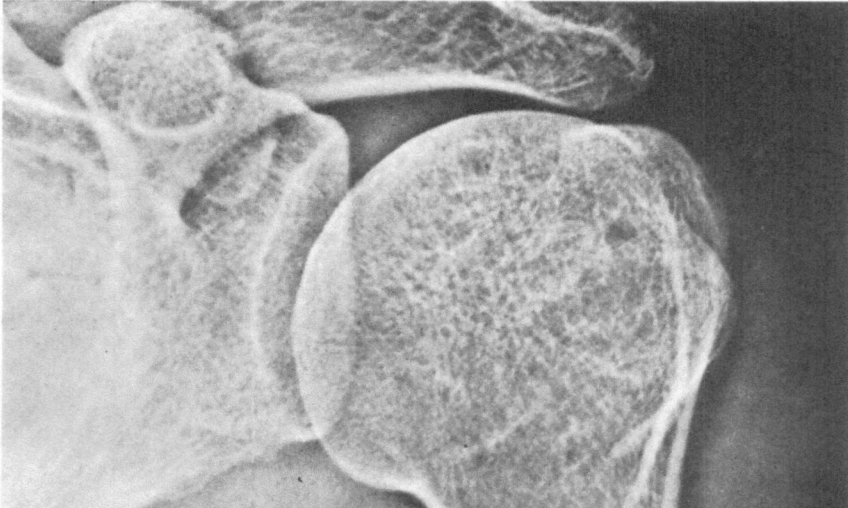

63/b

Fig. 63. H. S., 30 years, haemophilia B

(a, b) Right shoulder: marked humerus varus, destroyed joint surfaces, extensive cystic rarefaction, otherwise chronic atrophy. Left shoulder: acute haemarthrosis, the joint space is slightly open proximally. Intact articular surfaces. Sporadic small cysts in the head of the humerus

126

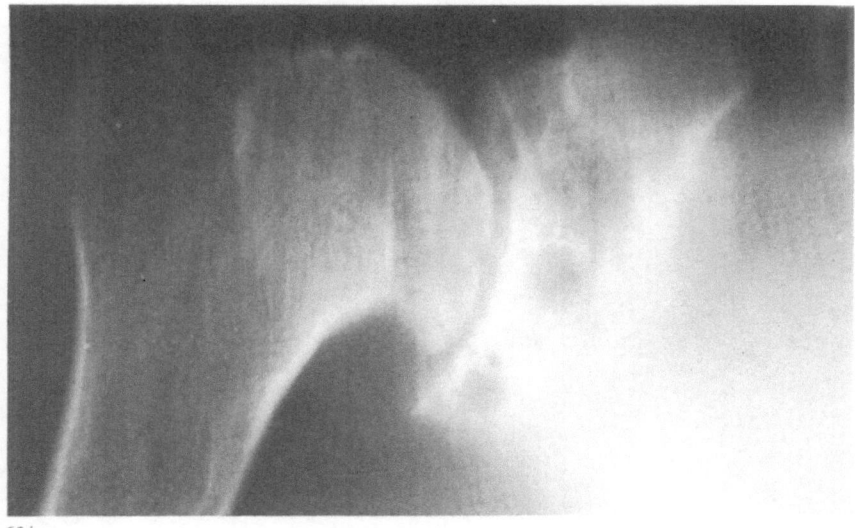

63/c

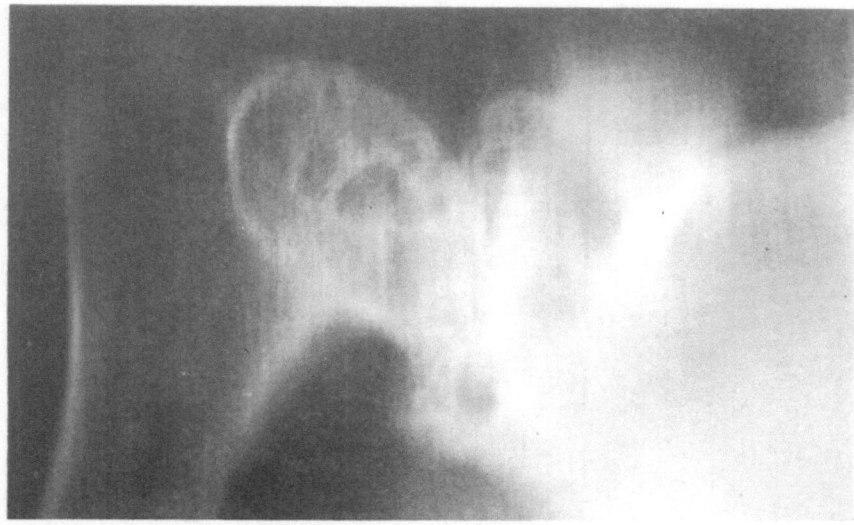

63/d

(c, d) Tomograms of the right shoulder. The joint space is markedly narrowed; irregular articular surfaces, nut-sized cysts behind the glenoid fossa and in the humeral epiphysis. The alterations visible on the right side remind of syringomyelia

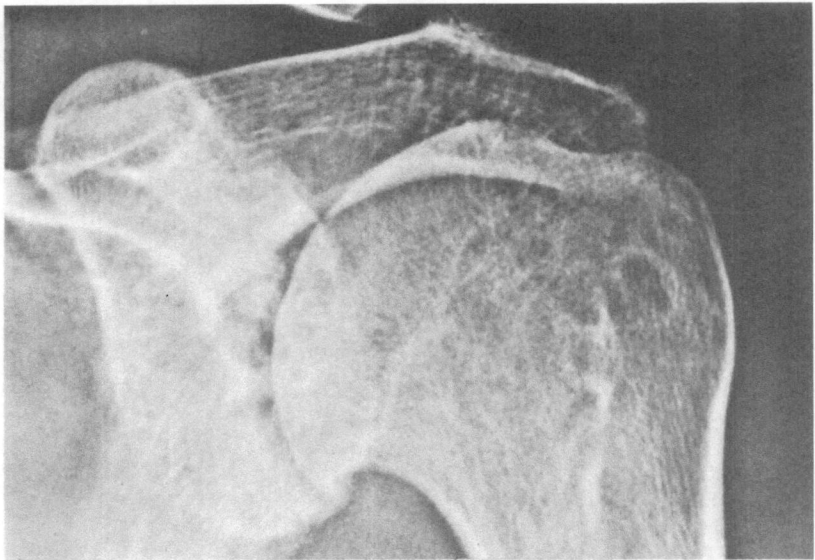

64/a

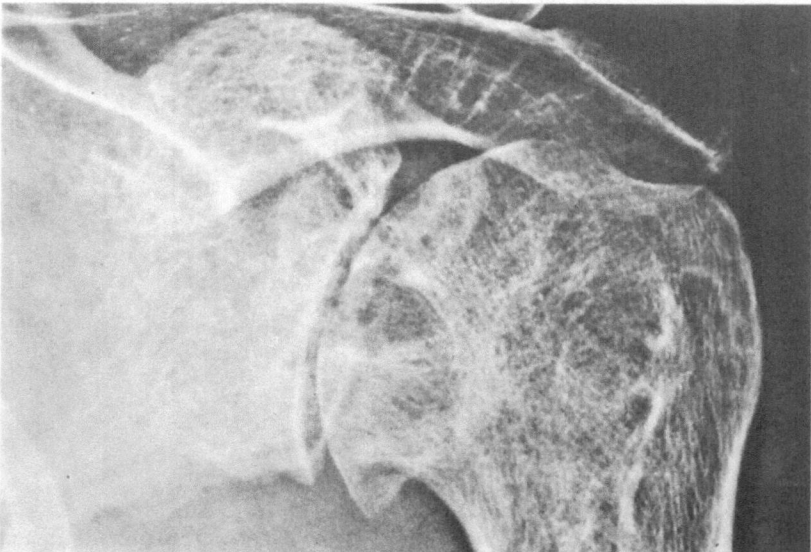

64/b

Fig. 64. S. J., haemophilia A

(a) At 23 years of age. The articular surface of the humerus is slightly irregular with randomly distributed cysts

(b) At 25 years of age. A significant advance of the process is notable: at the middle of the humeral joint surface the contour has disappeared over a section of 1 cm; under this defect a peanut-sized rarefaction is seen. Many cysts have formed. Chronic atrophy of the bones. The distal crest of the humeral articular surface is considerably elongated. Marked humerus varus

Wrist

Haemarthrosis

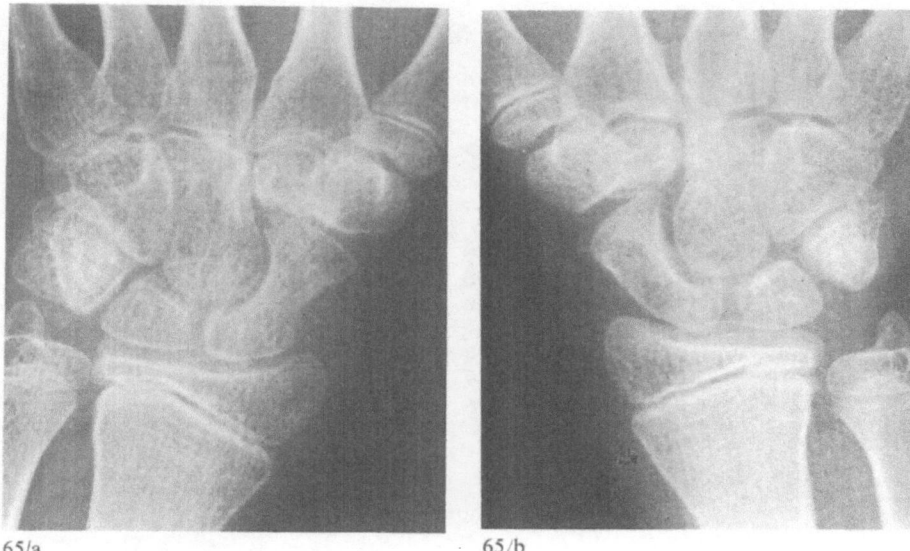

65/a   65/b

Fig. 65. D. V., 17 years, haemophilia A

(a, b) Recurrent episodes of haemarthrosis. On the comparative picture the bones of the left wrist are porotic. Intact articulations. The epiphysis of the radius is somewhat overdeveloped On the radial contour of the scaphoid bone an arched, sharp-bordered excavation indicates. bone resorption

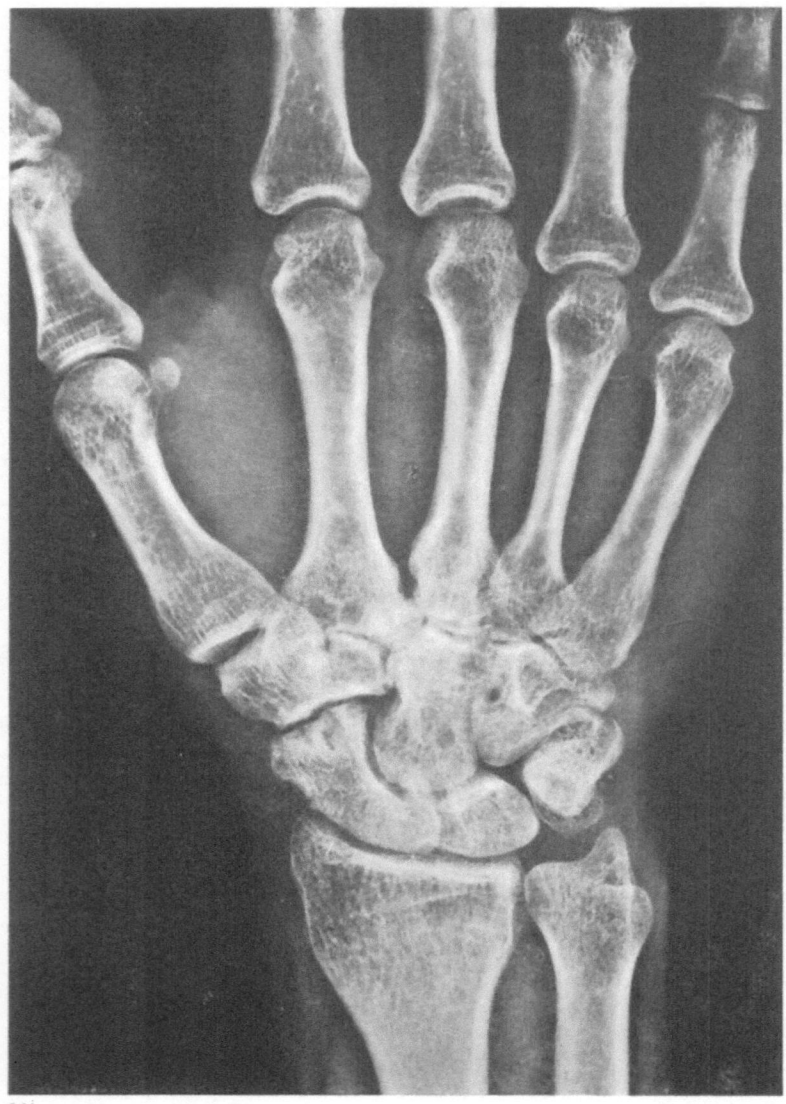

66/a

Fig. 66. B. J., 37 years, haemophilia A

(a–d) Lentil-sized cysts on the carpal bones and on the base of the 2nd meta-carpal bone. Coarse arthrosis in the articulation between the scaphoid and the two multangular bones, and in the carpometacarpal articulations

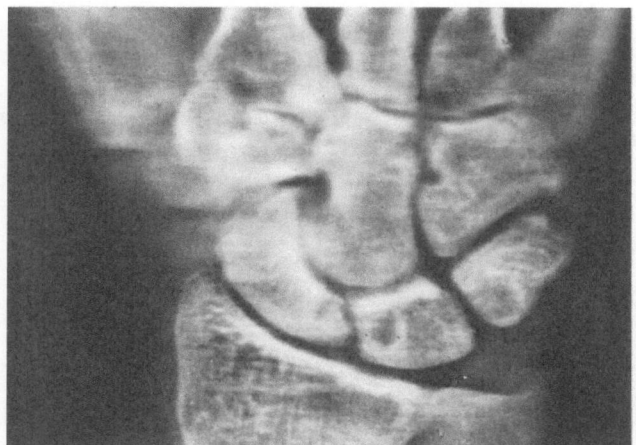

66/b

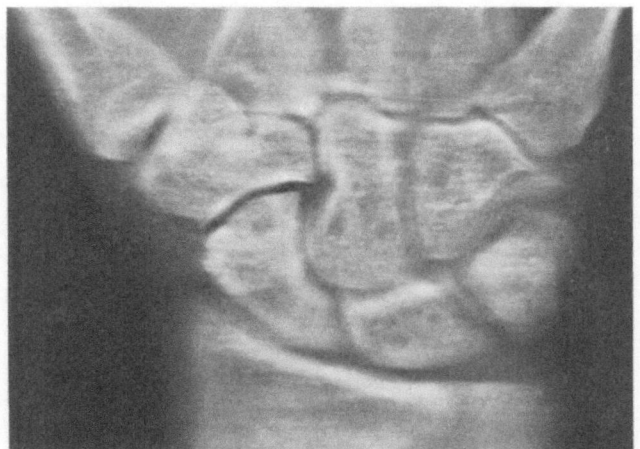

66/c

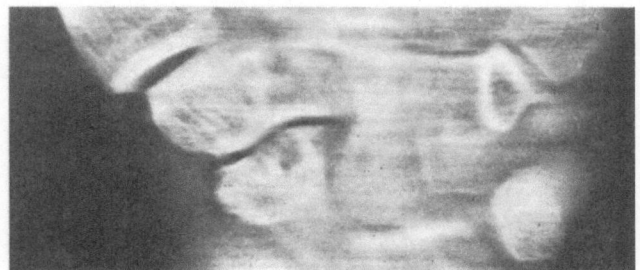

66/d

Non-Arthropathic Changes in Haemophiliacs

Fig. 67. B. I., 18 years, haemo-philia A

A peanut-sized round transparent area—an accessory bone in chondrous state: os centrale carpi—impacted between the capitate bone, the lesser multangular and the scaphoid bones. Advanced haemophilic arthropathy between the greater multangular bone and the 2nd metacarpal bone. Cartilaginous os centrale carpi occurs more frequently in haemophiliacs than in other patients

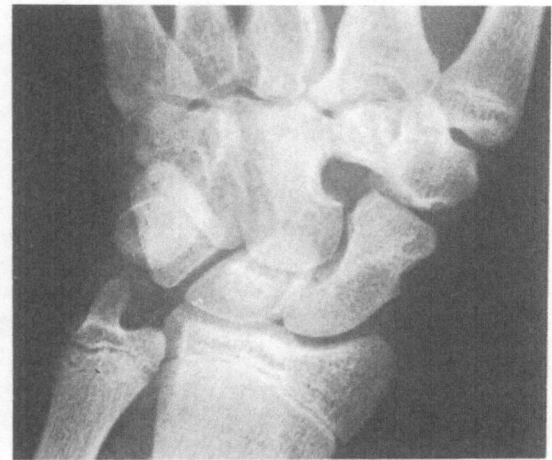

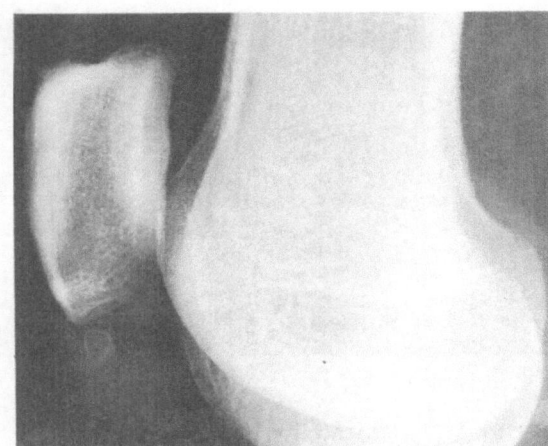

Fig. 68. P. F., 47 years, haemo-philia A

Squared off patella, persistent apophysis of the apex patellae

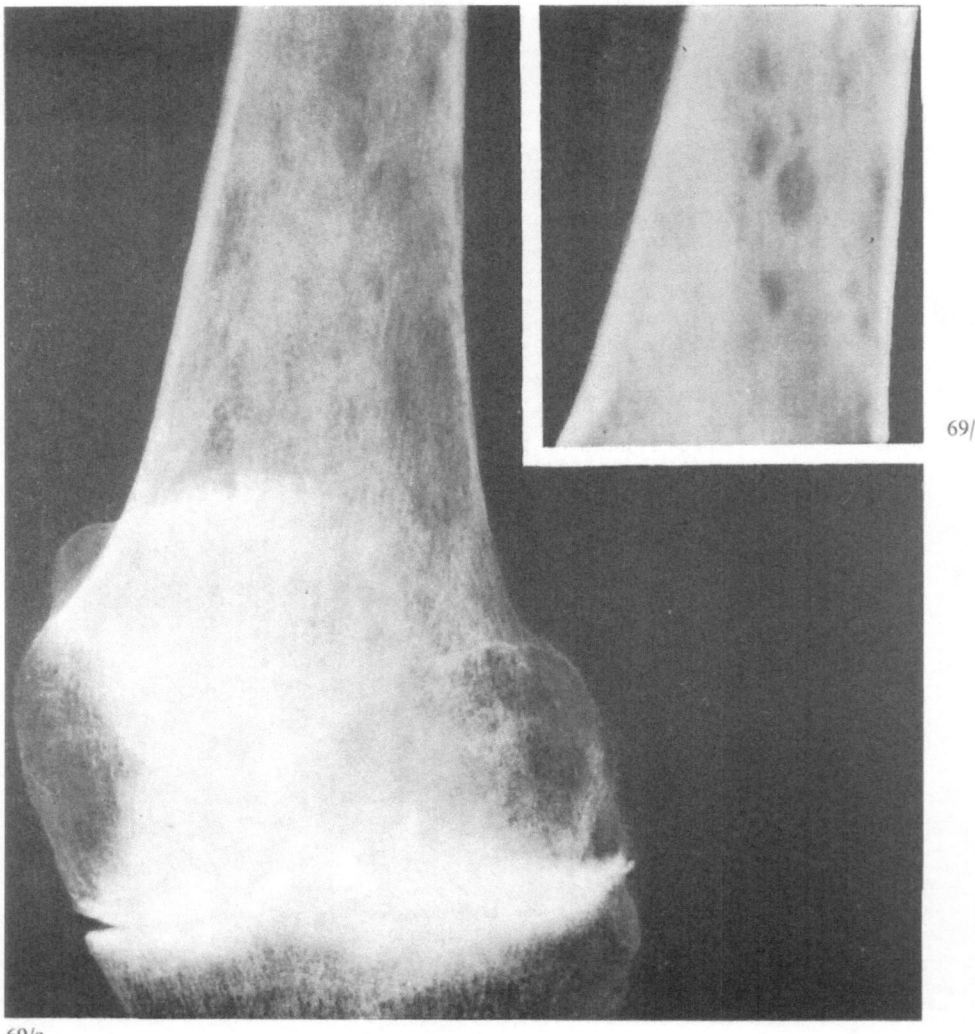

69/b

69/a

Fig. 69. M. J., 70 years, haemophilia A

(a, b) Regressive stage of pronounced haemophilic arthropathy. Numerous lentil- to pea-sized haemorrhagic cysts in the distal third of the femoral diaphysis without sclerotic demarcation. The cysts are particularly well visible on the tomogram (b)

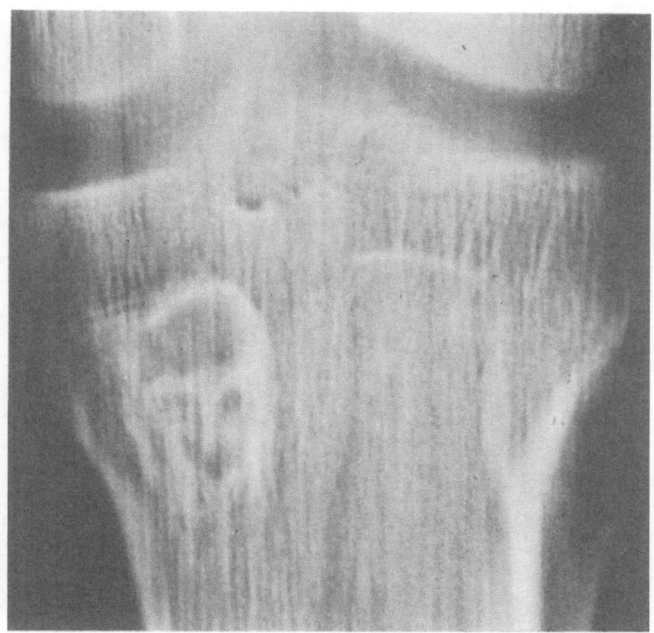

Fig. 70. T. I., 21 years, a patient without haemophilia

The tomogram displays a cystic rarefaction bordered by a coarse sclerosis in the medial half of the proximal metaphysis of the tibia. The alteration is characteristic of non-ossifying bone fibroma. This disease is differentiated from the above alteration shown in Fig. 69 by the typical sclerotic borderline of the cysts

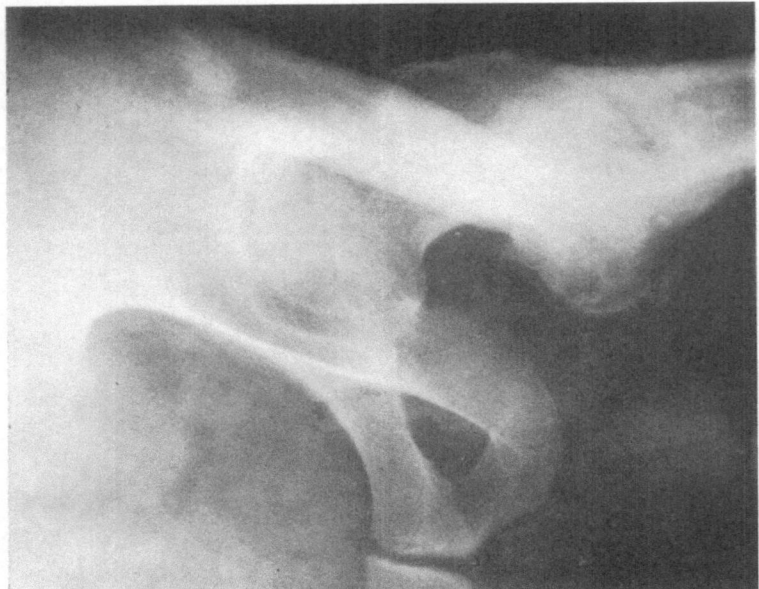

71/a

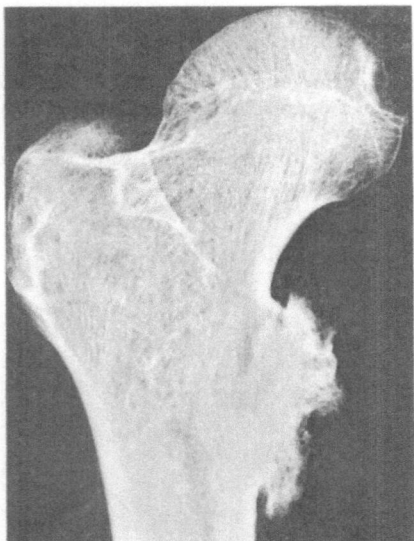

71/b

Fig. 71. P. S., 41 years, haemophilia A

(a) Extreme disposition of haemophiliacs to myositis ossificans. In the place of an earlier haemorrhage a tubular bone-like formation tends from the left anterior superior iliac spine to the lesser trochanter. The alteration is ossification of the iliacus muscle

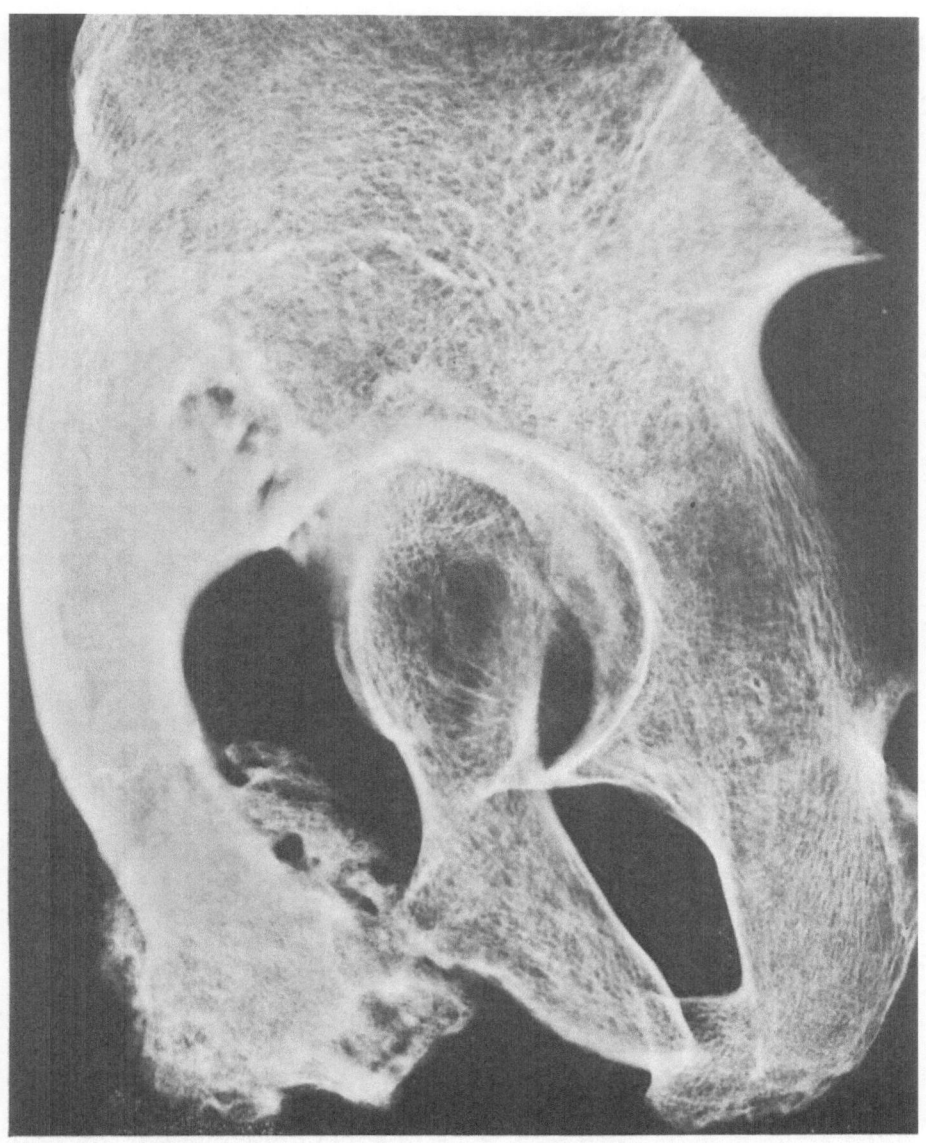

71/c

(b, c) Postmortem specimens. On the lesser trochanter at the site of insertion the bone substance is frayed and flattened, as the movement of the hip has inhibited complete ossification

137

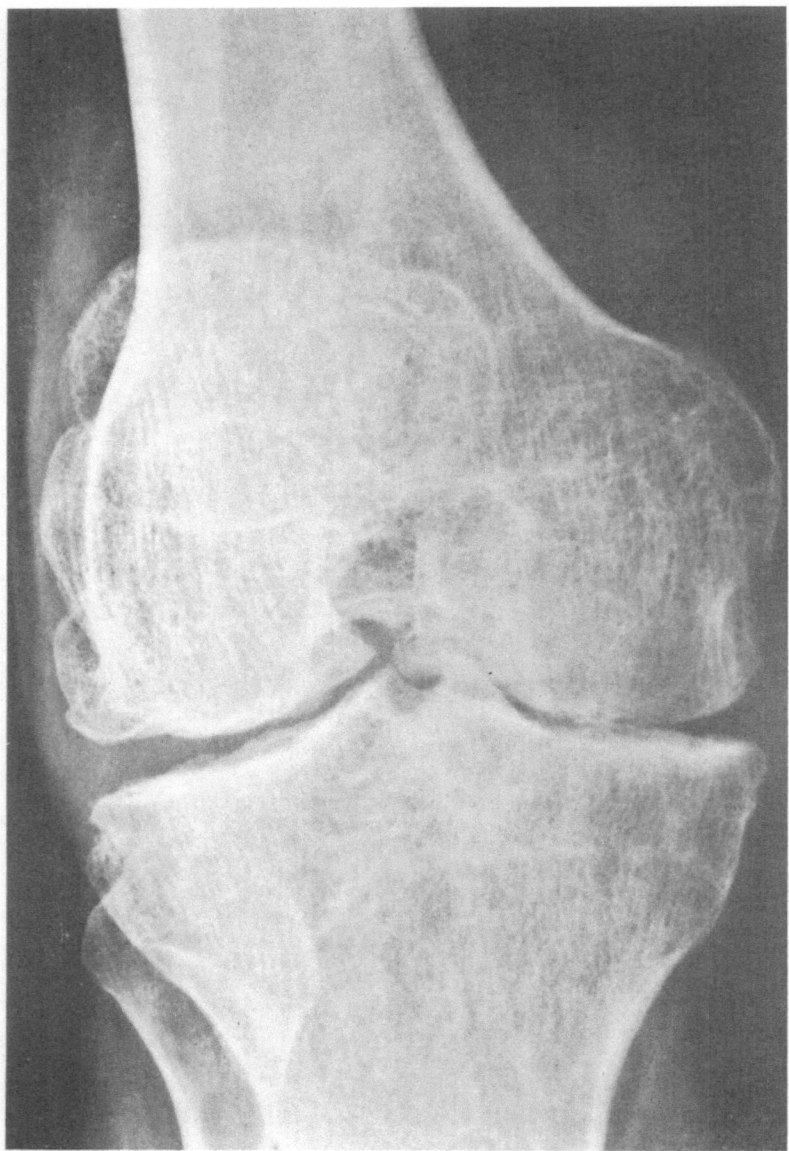

72/a

Fig. 72. S. J., 30 years, haemophilia B

(a–d) Comparative A–P and laterial view of knees. Regressive stage of haemophilic arthropathy in both knees. Fractures often occur in haemophiliacs. Coarsely impacted transversal fracture in the distal metaphysis of the left femur with formation of pseudoarticulation. Note the coarse bone apposition above the fracture, on the lateral contour

138

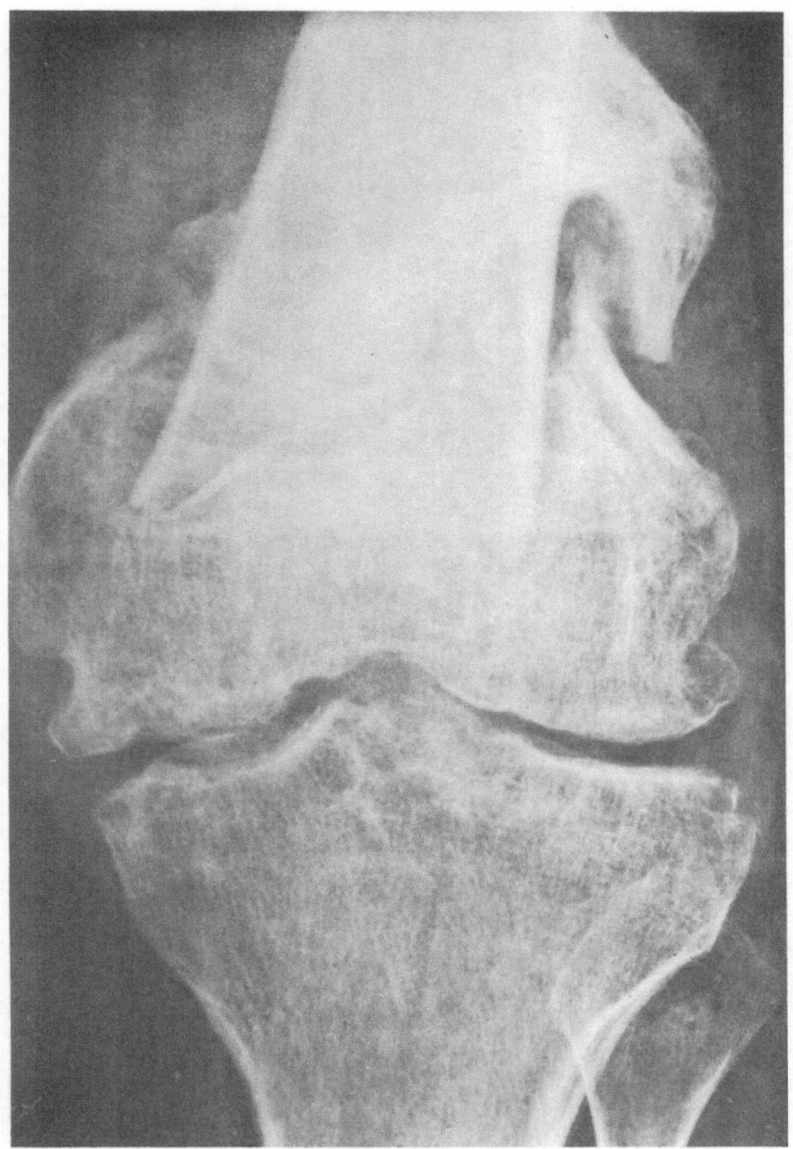

72/b

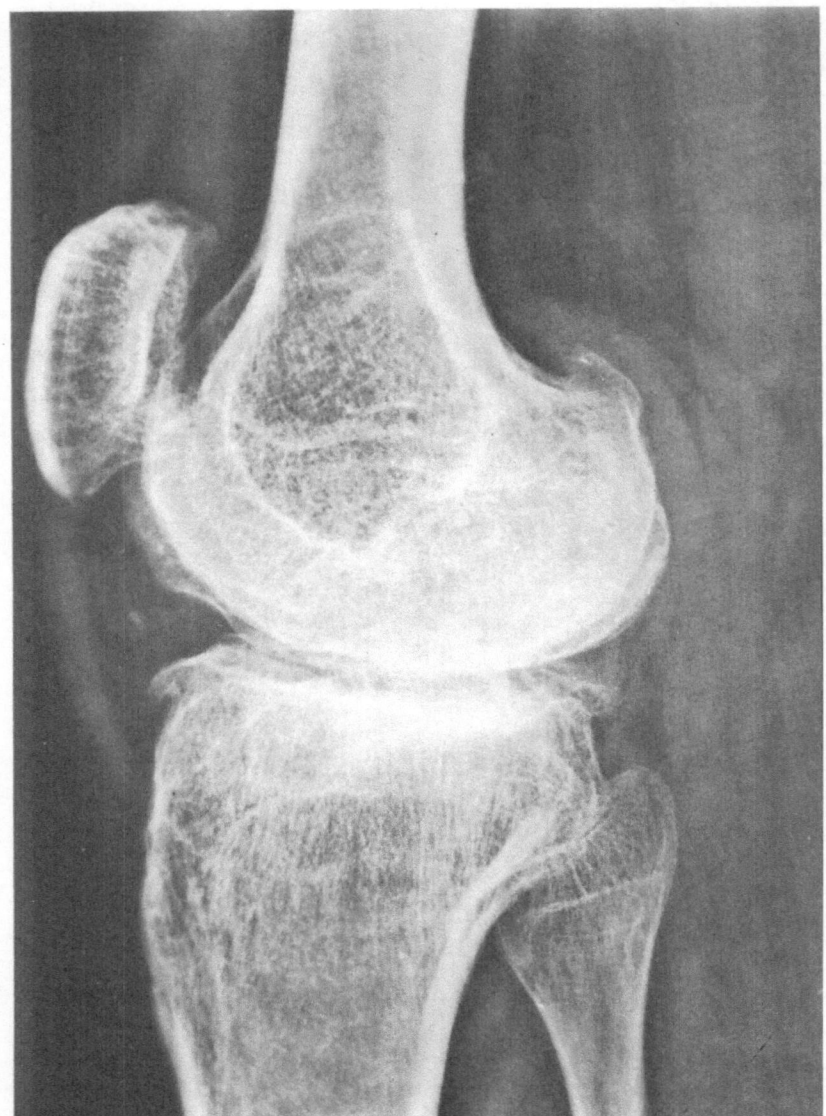

72/c

Fig. 72

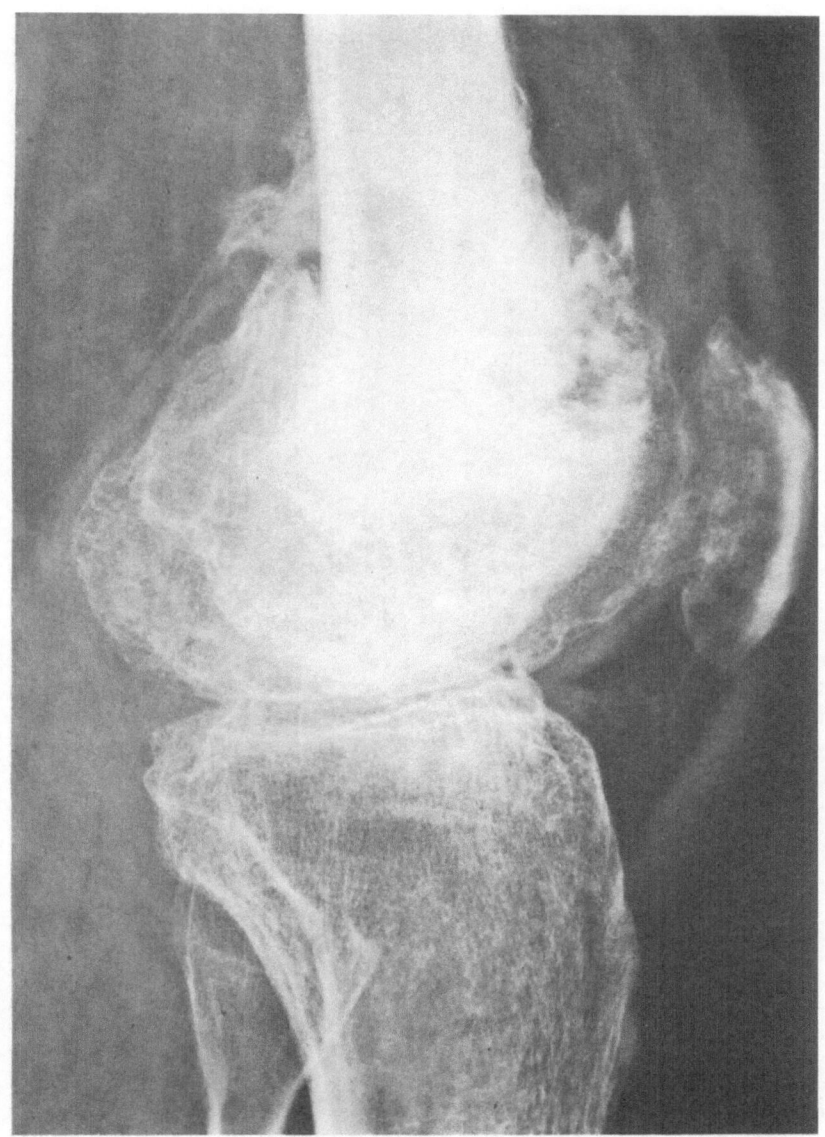

72/d

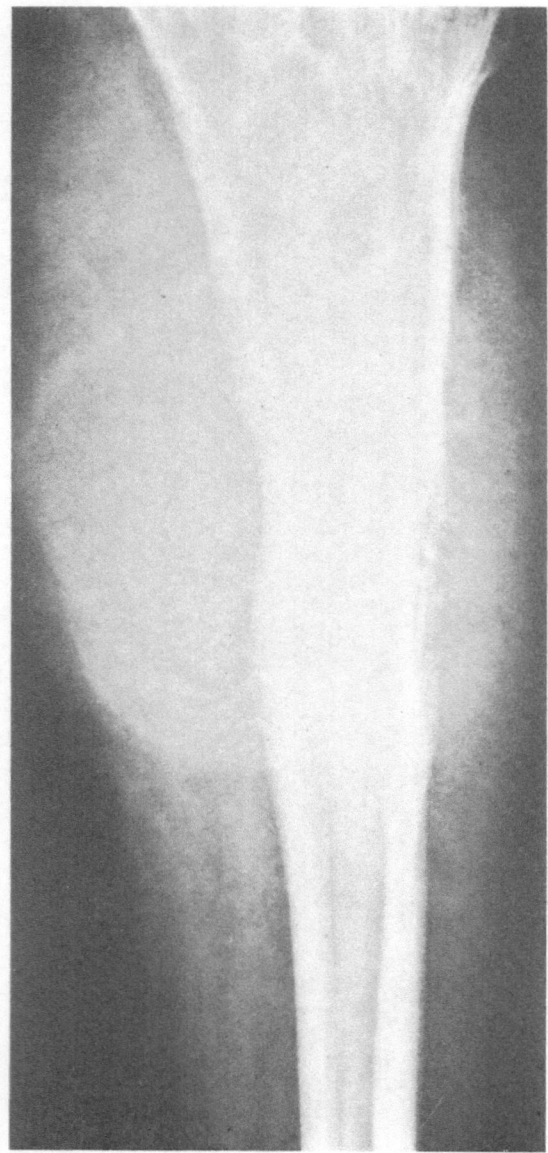

73/a

Fig. 73. Zs. L., 18 years, haemophilia A

(a, b) A–P and lateral views of
crural bones. Fist-sized organized
haematoma in the proximal part
of the leg; coarse resorption and
ossification in the tibia; extensive
destruction, bone resorption, and
pathological fracture of the fibula

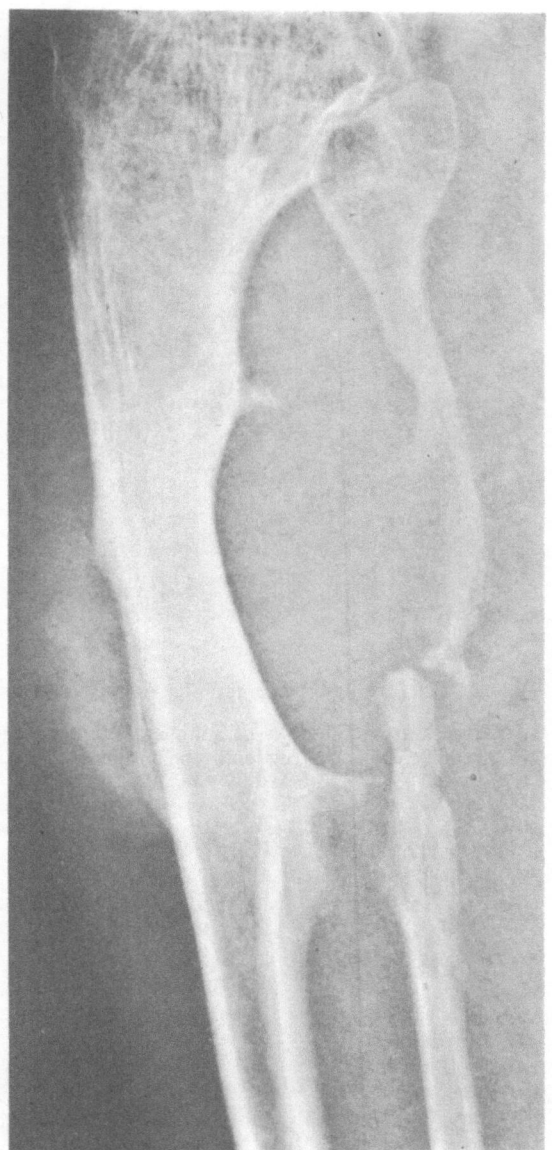

73/b

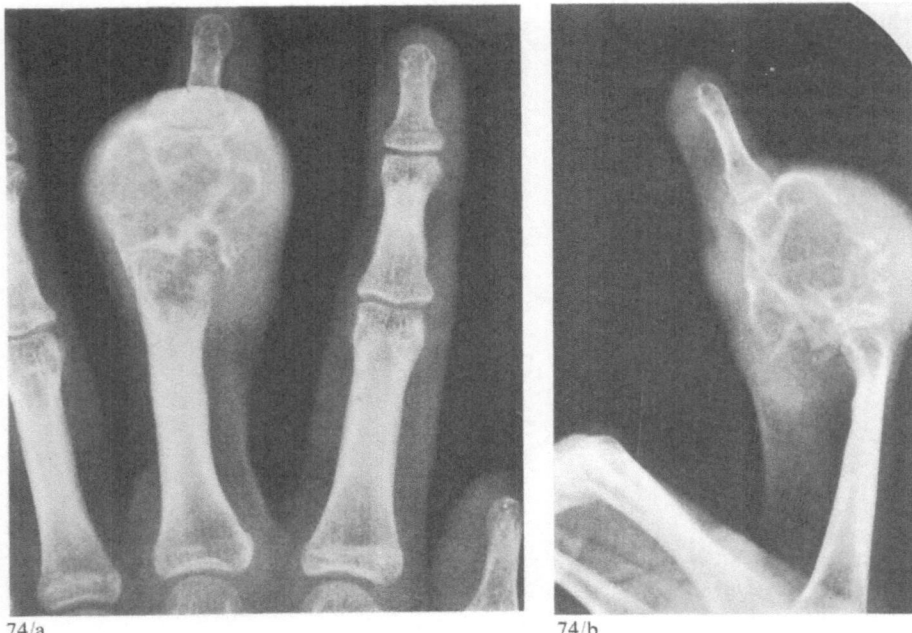

74/a   74/b

Fig. 74. Zs. L., 16 years, haemophilia A

(a, b) A–P and lateral views of a finger. Characteristic intraosteal expansive cystic pseudo-tumour and cortical destruction in the middle phalanx

144

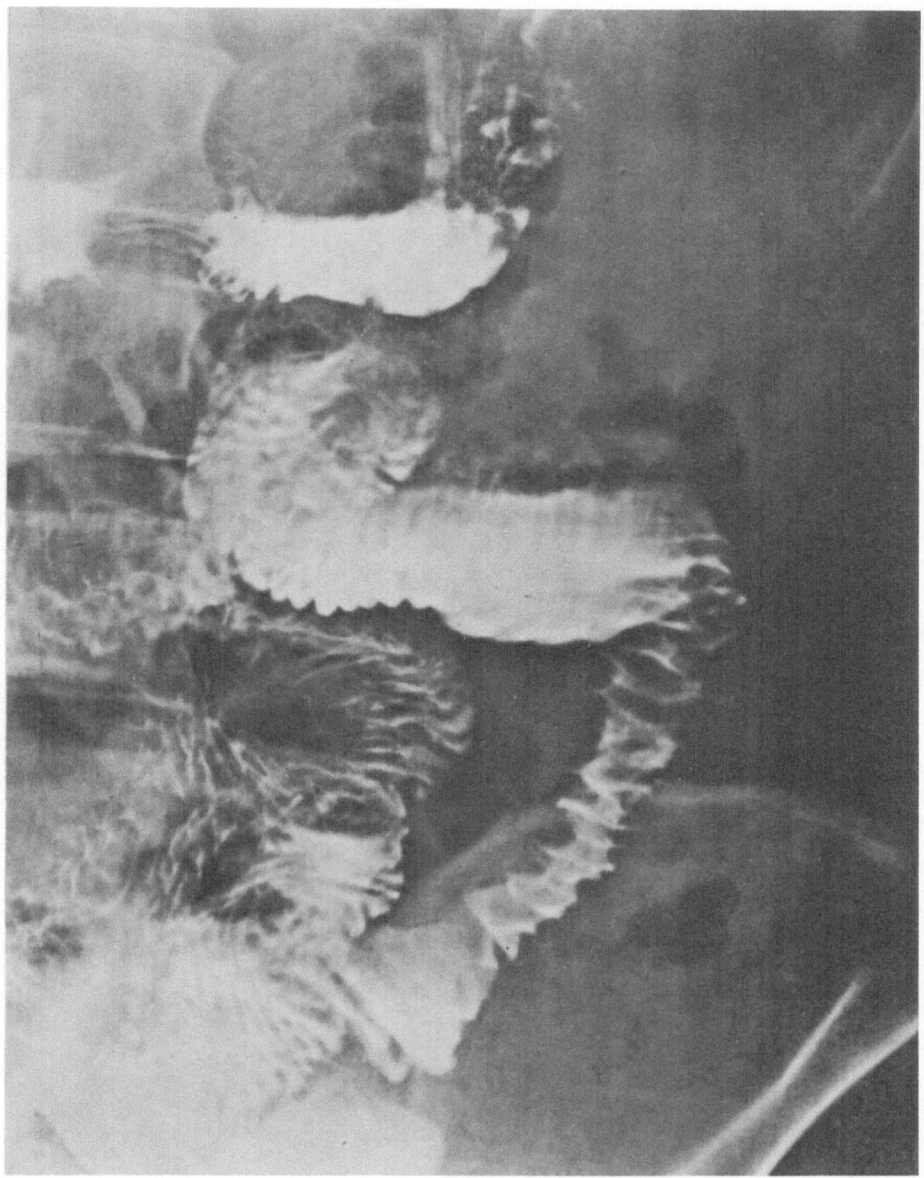

Fig. 75. P. Gy., 25 years, haemophilia A

Jejunal haematoma. Ileal loop with narrow lumen and irregular haustration situated at a distance, due to haematoma in the intestinal wall